P9-DEM-834

ALLERGIES
What You Need to Know

Johns Hopkins Editors

N. Franklin Adkinson, Jr., M.D.
Professor of Medicine
The Johns Hopkins University School of Medicine

Karen Huss, D.N.Sc.
Associate Professor of Nursing
The Johns Hopkins University School of Nursing

Jonathan Samet, M.D.
Professor and Chair, Epidemiology
The Johns Hopkins University School of Hygiene and Public Health

Editorial Director
Laura J. Wallace

Writer
Mark Giuliucci

Johns Hopkins Office of Consumer Health Information
Ron Sauder, Director
Molly L. Mullen, Editor

Johns Hopkins USA assists out-of-town patients with any aspect of arranging a visit to the Johns Hopkins Medical Institutions—from scheduling appointments to providing guidance on hotels, transportation, and preferred routes of travel. The program has up-to-date information on clinical practices and is a resource center for maps, visitor guides, and other materials of interest to non-local patients. Client Services Coordinators in the Johns Hopkins USA offices are available Monday through Friday from 8:30 a.m. until 5:00 p.m. (Eastern). They can be reached toll-free at 1-800-507-9952 or locally at 410-614-USA1. You can also visit Johns Hopkins on the World Wide Web at *http://hopkins.med.jhu.edu/*.

Johns Hopkins
HEALTH

ALLERGIES
What You Need to Know

TIME
LIFE
BOOKS

Alexandria, Virginia

The information in this book is for your general knowledge only. It is not intended as a substitute for the advice of a physician. You should seek prompt medical care for any specific health problems you may have.

TIME ®
LIFE
BOOKS

Time-Life Books is a division of Time Life Inc.

Time Life Inc.
President and CEO: George Artandi

Time-Life Custom Publishing
Vice President and Publisher: Terry Newell
Vice President of Sales and Marketing: Neil Levin
Director of Special Sales: Liz Ziehl
Editor for Special Markets: Anna Burgard

© 1999 The Johns Hopkins University
All rights reserved.
Published by Ottenheimer Publishers, Inc.
5 Park Center Court, Suite 300
Owings Mills, MD 21117-5001
JH006M L K J I H G F E D C B A

No part of this book may be reproduced in any form or by any electronic or mechanical means, including information storage and retrieval devices or systems, without prior written permission from the publisher, except that brief passages may be quoted for reviews.

First printing. Printed and bound in U.S.A. M L K J I H G F E D C B A

Time-Life is a trademark of Time Warner Inc. U.S.A.

ISBN: 0-7370-1609-4

Library of Congress Cataloging-in-Publication Data
Giuliucci, Mark.
       Allergies : what you need to know / by Mark Giuliucci.
              p.   cm. — (Johns Hopkins health)
       ISBN 0-7370-1609-4 (pbk. : alk. paper)
       1. Allergy Popular works.   I. Title.   II. Series.
RC584.G   1999
616.97—dc21   99-26955
                                                             CIP

Books produced by Time-Life Custom Publishing are available at special bulk discounts for promotional and premium use. Custom adaptations can also be created to meet your specific marketing goals. Call 1-800-323-5255.

CONTENTS

INTRODUCTION

What's the worst thing about allergies? It depends on whom you ask. People with hay fever can't stand the runny nose and the itchy eyes. Folks with food allergies despise those red, swollen hives. Kids with asthma dread sudden attacks that can steal their breath for hours or days at a time.

But the worst part about allergies isn't the symptoms they cause. It's this simple fact: Allergic reactions are completely unnecessary. Medically speaking, they serve no useful purpose. They don't protect you from viruses, heart disease, or infections. They're just a misguided reaction to a harmless little piece of protein that you happen to eat, breathe, or touch.

Allergies may be a biological "mistake," but they're nothing to sneeze at. Each year, Americans with hay fever spend about $3.5 billion on doctors' bills and medications. Asthma may add another $6.2 billion to the total. Allergies and other nasal problems are the second most common reason—after dental care—that people visit the doctor.

If you suffer from constant or severe allergic symptoms, there are probably times you'd rather have your teeth drilled. Allergy symptoms range from the mildly irritating, like poison ivy rashes, to the deadly serious, like anaphylactic shock caused by insect stings or food reactions. For people allergic to dust, mold, or pets, symptoms can last year-round.

Fortunately, there's growing hope for allergy sufferers. Allergic reactions are unnecessary and so are the symptoms. With a little work and a little patience, you can learn to control your allergies and regain control of your life.

The first—and best—of these strategies is avoidance. Simply put, what you don't touch can't hurt you. Once you and your doctor discover what you're allergic to, you'll be able to take a number of practical steps to keep away from your "triggers." These can range from reading food labels to planting "sneezeless" plants in your garden. Sure, it's going to take a little work. But the results will be more than worth it.

No matter how hard you try, however, there will be times when allergies sneak up on you. That's when it's time for the second strategy: medication. There are many medicines on the market today that can help combat—and even prevent—allergic reactions.

The last line of defense is immunotherapy injections, or "allergy shots." In many cases, it's possible to build up tolerance to your allergies through a series of shots that contain tiny amounts of the protein that causes your reactions. This can be a long process. You may need months or even years of injections to build up your immunity. But if you simply can't avoid your allergy triggers, immunotherapy is the closest thing to a sure bet against symptoms.

The future holds great promise. Scientists are closing in on a number of treatments that may prove quicker and more effective than immunotherapy. Some involve shots that contain synthetic versions of those allergy-causing proteins. Others seek to block the antibodies in your immune system that spot the allergy proteins and start the reaction process. Still others focus on stopping the release of the immune-system chemicals that cause the symptoms of allergies. Some researchers believe that one day it may be possible to write off allergies completely. Imagine that: a world without sneezes, wheezes, hives, and runny noses!

For now, however, it's going to take a little more effort. The major players in the battle against allergies will be your family doctor, your allergist, and you. It's going to be a partnership, but you will need to take charge. You will have to remember to take your medication. And you may have to change your routines—everything from house cleaning to exercising—to help keep your allergies at bay.

The Johns Hopkins University (including its world-renowned schools of medicine, nursing, and public health) and the closely related Johns Hopkins Health System are well known for their commitment to medical research, education and patient care. For the past eight years, The Johns Hopkins Hospital has been ranked as the number one hospital in the United States in an annual survey conducted by *U.S. News and World Report*.

In this book, Johns Hopkins presents a comprehensive, clearly written guide to the challenge of life with allergies. When it comes to health advice, you want expert knowledge and compassionate guidance, and that's precisely what you'll find here. The information in this book is based on the latest research and years of experience of the finest health professionals anywhere. You can be assured that what you read within these pages is information you can trust and just what you need at your side in your fight against allergies.

If you have always believed that allergies or asthma is inevitable, it's time for a new approach. You can greatly improve the quality of your life. You're not doomed to a life of nasal congestion or asthma attacks. Your life can be normal again.

Let's get started on the road to breathing easy!

CHAPTER 1

The Allergic Reaction: Sneezes, Wheezes, and More

At this very moment, even as you settle down on your sofa to read this book, your body is under attack—from bacteria, viruses, and other nasty microscopic critters. They're trying to sneak under your skin and do their dirty work. They're looking for any opening they can slip through—your nose, mouth, ears, even a little paper cut on your finger.

It's enough to make you want to jump up and take a shower. But in truth, it's no big deal. Every minute of every day, your body's immune system is hard at work spotting would-be invaders and crushing them before they do any harm. Every so often a cold or flu virus may slip past the guards and set up shop for a while. For the most part, though, things stay under control unless there's something seriously wrong with your immune system.

As terrific as our bodies' defenders are, they make mistakes on occasion. They're so used to warding off bad guys that they sometimes shoot first and ask questions later. That's how it is with allergies. When a foreign protein gets inside, your immune system thinks it's found an enemy and unleashes its whole arsenal on it—and you start feeling the effects. Your nose runs. Your eyes water. You sneeze. You wheeze. Sometimes you get sick to your stomach. In very serious cases, you may have trouble breathing.

All this for no good reason. The thing that caused your allergic reaction may have been nothing more than an innocent little mold spore or a bit of pollen. One minute it's floating gently through the air, looking for a soft place to land. The next minute it's getting hammered by your body's full battalion of killer immune cells. It's really a giant waste of effort, and you pay the price.

In this chapter, we'll explain exactly how allergic reactions happen. We'll take a closer look at your immune system so you can understand what happens when it kicks into gear. We'll talk about who is most likely to get allergies. And we'll touch briefly on the different kinds of allergies, from those that affect your skin to those that stuff up your sinuses.

In later chapters we'll show you ways to stop allergies. There's no need to surrender to sneezes and sniffles anymore. You and your doctor can work together to relieve your allergy problems, even if you've been struggling with them for years. We'll show you scores of things you can try—from changing your pillows or vacuum cleaner to taking modern allergy medications that can ease your symptoms.

THE WEAPONS OF DEFENSE

The main players in your body's immune system are white blood cells. Your body makes many different kinds, from giant, enemy-eating macrophages to "killer" T cells that wipe out invaders. They're working 24 hours a day to spot and destroy **antigens**—things like viruses, bacteria, and parasites. While all this may sound a little scary, that's how things go inside your body. You've got to get the bad guys before they get you.

The white blood cells we're going to pay the most attention to right now are called **lymphocytes**. They're made in the marrow of your bones and are stored in specific parts of your body until they're needed. Your body creates so many lymphocytes that they'd be hard to count without a supercomputer. You may have 2,000,000,000,000—two trillion—of them floating around at any given time.

There are two main types of lymphocytes: B cells and T cells. The T cells attack problems head-on by destroying body cells that have been infected or damaged by antigens. B cells, on the other hand, do their job in a more roundabout way. They gather in lymph nodes and other immunity-related organs like the spleen, tonsils, and appendix. When an antigen shows up in the body, B cells create special proteins called **antibodies**. These antibodies attach themselves to antigens. Once an antibody hooks on to the antigen, the antigen is unable to function normally. If it's a virus, the antibody makes it unable to enter a body cell and reproduce. If it's a bacterium, the antibody prevents it from spreading its toxic effects.

Antibodies are highly specialized; they react only to specific antigens. If a flu virus enters your body, only "flu antibodies" go to work. The others continue patrolling, looking for their special antigens. Every time you're exposed to a new antigen, the body creates antibodies specially designed to fight it. And once an antibody is created, it sticks around for a long time—sometimes for life. This is why the immune system is said to have a memory. When you get chicken pox, for example, your body makes specific antibodies. After you get better, some of these antibodies stick around in the body for years. That way, if the chicken pox virus shows up again, even decades later, your body is already prepared to fight it—and you won't get sick again.

GOING OVERBOARD

What does all this have to do with allergies? Well, as we've said, sometimes your immune system gets confused. It sees a harmless substance in the body—pet dander, mold, or pollen, for example—and mistakes it for a dangerous foreign substance. These usually tame substances are called **allergens**, which are often an animal or plant protein.

When your immune system spies an allergen, it unleashes specialized antibodies that bind onto the invader. These antibodies, made of a substance called **immunoglobulin E (IgE)**, are themselves attached to the outside of larger cells. So now we have three things all tied together: the allergen, the IgE antibody, and the bigger cells, which are called **mast cells** and **basophils**. Each mast cell or basophil may hold tens of thousands of IgE antibodies in special receptors on its outer wall.

HOW SYMPTOMS HAPPEN

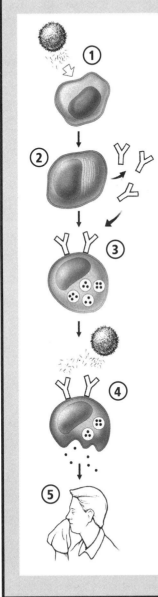

The main players in the allergic reaction are mast cells or basophils. These are giant storehouses of chemicals that are used to fight foreign substances in your body. Here's how they get triggered to release their load.

1. When an allergen such as ragweed pollen enters the body for the first time, it encounters a B cell, part of your immune system.

2. The B cell creates a huge number of antibodies that are designed specifically to identify the allergen (in this case, ragweed pollen).

3. The antibodies attach themselves to mast cells or basophils.

4. When the allergen enters the body a second time, the antibodies grab hold of it. This triggers the mast cell or basophil to release its load of chemicals, the most important of which is histamine.

5. Chemicals from the mast cell or basophil cause allergic symptoms ranging from sneezing to itching.

What happens next is pretty explosive. When enough IgE antibodies grab on to allergens, the mast cell or basophil literally opens up and releases its payload, which consists of granules of killer chemicals, the most important of which are called **histamines.** Histamines cause your body to react in several ways. First, they can cause smooth muscles in your lungs, stomach lining, and other places to contract. Second, they cause your blood vessels to open wide, allowing blood to flow more easily through the body. Finally, they make it easier for fluid (containing more immune-system chemicals) to pass from the bloodstream into individual cells. This chain of events is called the **allergic inflammatory response.**

While this inflammation is an effective way to fight unfriendly invaders, it's completely unnecessary against harmless antigens. All you get are the side effects. Some, like a runny nose, hives, or diarrhea, are merely uncomfortable. Others can be much more serious. Asthma is usually caused by allergens. Some estimate that 50 percent of adults and more than 80 percent of children with asthma have some associated allergic sensitivities. In some people, breathing in an allergen like pollen or pet dander causes the air passages in the lungs to narrow and fill with mucus and inflammatory cells. This can make breathing extremely difficult. You wheeze and cough and feel a terrible tightness in your chest. Asthma attacks can last for minutes, hours, or even days, and they're very scary for those who suffer from the disease.

A condition called anaphylaxis can be even worse. It usually begins within moments of being exposed to an allergen. Unlike most allergic reactions, anaphylaxis

WHO'S AT RISK FOR ALLERGIES?

Nearly 45 million Americans have allergies. That's an incredibly high number; it means that one in six of us is susceptible.

Some people are more likely to have allergies than others. Heredity plays a big role. People may have a genetic tendency to produce greater amounts of IgE—the so-called allergy antibody. Unfortunately, this trait can be passed on from generation to generation, just like baldness, blue eyes, or blond hair.

In fact, if both your parents have allergies, you have a 60 percent chance of getting them, too. That's nearly four times the normal risk. If only one of your parents suffers from allergies, you have about a 30 percent chance. If neither Mom nor Dad has allergies, you have about a 10 percent chance of developing them. The really bad news about inheriting the ability to make lots of IgE is that it increases your chances of having many types of allergies, from hay fever to food allergies to asthma.

It's not only heredity that increases your risk. If you grew up in a household with smokers, you're more likely to develop certain allergies. Socioeconomic status seems to play a role, too; people from poor backgrounds may have a higher risk of getting some allergies than people from higher income families. Being exposed to allergens like molds, pollen, dust mites, pet dander, and certain foods can, over time, increase the likelihood of becoming allergic to them.

Even your early childhood is important. If you were a light baby—less than 5 1/2 pounds at birth—you may be more likely to develop allergies later. The same is true if you weren't breast-fed. If you were born during a high-pollen season, you may have a higher risk of getting hay fever as you grow older. If you had a family pet, you will be more likely to be allergic to dogs or cats later.

affects your whole body. You may break out in itchy hives. Your throat can swell, and the air passages in your lungs can close down. Your heart can start beating rapidly, and your blood pressure can drop. If you're not treated right away, severe cases of anaphylaxis can be fatal. Every year, hundreds of Americans die from anaphylaxis.

THE WORST OFFENDERS

When most people think about allergies, they focus on hay fever. That's understandable, since it's by far the most common type of allergy. But everything from latex gloves to bee stings can cause allergic reactions, too. In fact, there's a whole world of allergies to deal with. We'll touch on each of the major categories in later chapters. For now, here's a quick summary.

Hay fever. The medical term for this is allergic rhinitis. It's caused by allergens that you breathe and produces a number of unpleasant symptoms—sneezing, runny nose, itchy eyes, nasal congestion, and more.

There are two major types of allergic rhinitis: seasonal and perennial. With seasonal rhinitis, you get allergic reactions during specific times of the year. When pollen counts are high, for example, or when there's lots of mold in the air, seasonal allergies are at their worst.

With perennial rhinitis, however, the problem can exist all year long. That's because the allergen that you're allergic to never goes away. For example, microscopic parasites called dust mites live in your house 365 days a year, and their excretions can cause the same reactions in some people as pollen or mold. Other people are very sensitive to pet dander, the tiny bits of skin that dogs and cats (and humans) shed all the time. For some folks, things get even more distasteful. Saliva and secretions from insects—especially mosquitoes and cockroaches—also can cause allergic reactions.

The good thing about allergic rhinitis is that it can usually be controlled. If something in your house is causing the problem, you usually can eliminate or lessen your exposure—by spending a little less time with your pets, for example, or reducing the amount of mold or pollen that gets indoors.

Asthma. This condition affects 14 million to 15 million Americans and is especially common in children. Although the exact cause of asthma is unknown, it's very closely related to allergies and is probably genetic in many cases. Many things that cause hay fever—like pet dander, mold, and pollen—can trigger an asthma attack. When this happens, the passageways in the lungs swell up and narrow. At the same time they fill with mucus. This combination can make breathing extremely difficult.

Fortunately, the right combination of allergen avoidance and medication can control asthma. While it's a serious disease, it doesn't mean the end of your active lifestyle.

Food allergies. Nothing is worse than having a bad reaction to a good dinner. Food allergies can be serious, causing symptoms such as stomach cramps, nausea, diarrhea, vomiting, hives, wheezing, and even asthma attacks. But true food allergies are actually quite rare. Most people who have had unpleasant reactions either ate contaminated food or have a food intolerance, meaning they ate something their bodies can't digest very well. While "food poisoning" and food intolerances can result in nasty symptoms, they are not caused by the release of histamine in the body and so aren't related to allergies.

But some people are allergic to certain foods. Most food allergies are caused by proteins found in peanuts, wheat, soybean products, egg whites, and cow's milk. Food allergies are usually diagnosed by lab tests or an "elimination diet," in which you give up certain foods to see if things get better.

Drug allergies. The most common drug allergy is to penicillin, but there is a whole range of drugs that can cause allergic reactions in some people. These include some types of anticonvulsant medications, insulin, and local anesthetics. As with foods, most drug reactions aren't really due to allergies. Nearly one million people don't tolerate aspirin well, for instance. While they may develop allergy-like symptoms, such as hives and wheezing, there's no allergic reaction taking place.

Most drug allergies are usually mild. A skin rash is the most common reaction, and it can be treated with common allergy medication. But things can get out of control sometimes, and some allergic reactions can be very dangerous. So it's smart to be aware of your drug allergies—and always make sure your doctor knows about them, too.

Insect bites and stings. For most of us, mosquito bites just itch and bee stings just, well, sting. But for 1 to 2 percent of Americans, insect bites or stings can have very serious consequences. They can cause severe allergic reactions, including deadly anaphylaxis. People who are allergic to insects usually carry emergency medication. A quick injection of epinephrine can fight off the allergic reaction before anaphylaxis occurs.

Contact dermatitis. Also called skin allergies, contact dermatitis occurs when you have a reaction after touching certain things. The most common type of contact dermatitis is caused by plants like poison ivy, poison oak, or poison sumac. These plants contain an oil that causes allergic reactions in millions of people.

Skin allergies aren't caused only by plants. Metals like nickel, which is often found in jewelry, can do it. So can latex used in gloves. And for some people, makeup, hair dyes, and even deodorants can cause skin rashes. Rashes from skin allergies are usually delayed; they don't show up for 24 to 48 hours after you touch the allergen.

Atopic dermatitis. Also known as eczema, this skin problem isn't really an allergic reaction. But 70 percent of people who get atopic dermatitis have a family history of respiratory or food allergies. About one-third of children with eczema will go on to develop hay fever and other respiratory allergies.

We've been talking about the most common allergies, but it's important to remember that almost any substance can cause allergies in some people. But respiratory allergies like hay fever are far and away the most common. So let's talk in detail about respiratory allergies. The story is a familiar one. It's a beautiful April day. The robins are chirping. The air is crisp. The dogwoods are blooming. You should be thinking thoughts of spring—but instead you're up to your watery eyes with hay fever. How do you fight back? In the next chapter, we'll show you how.

CHAPTER 2

Hay Fever: The Reason You're Sneezing

Breathe in, breathe out. Breathe in, breathe out. Most of the time we don't even think about it. We need oxygen to live, so we just take air in and let air out.

Sometimes, though, the air we breathe contains more than we bargain for. In the springtime, it carries tree pollen so fine that you can't even see it. In the summer and fall, grasses and other plants join the party. Then there's tiny stuff like dust mites, pet dander, and mold spores that linger all year round. All this gets pulled into your nose and lungs every time you draw a breath. And for nearly one in six Americans, it leads to a familiar sound: Aaaaa-chooo!

In this chapter, we're going to talk about airborne allergies, or allergic rhinitis. Airborne allergies are the most common of all allergies. And they can often be the toughest to avoid. But with a little planning and extra effort, you can help bring things under control—and start breathing easier.

HAY FEVER

The most common type of airborne allergy is hay fever. Actually, hay and fever have nothing to do with it. But it's easy to see where the term came from. In the old days, before tractors, combines, and reapers, most people in America worked and lived on farms. Hay was a common crop, used for animal feed. When it came time to harvest and bale the hay in late summer, great numbers of workers went into the fields. And many of them had runny noses, headaches, and sore throats. It seemed like a pretty straightforward connection—hay causes fevers.

Today we know better. Hay wasn't the culprit. It was pollen from all sorts of weeds, especially ragweed, that caused the reaction. (Pollen is the male part of the weed's reproductive cycle. It gets released when plants bloom and then drifts through the air in search of other plants to pollinate.) These weeds just happened to be in bloom at the same time as the hay. And what the workers developed wasn't a true fever, like that caused by flu. It was a severe allergic reaction.

Doctors today usually refer to hay fever as seasonal allergic rhinitis. The "seasonal" and "allergic" parts are pretty easy to understand. "Rhinitis" comes from the Greek words "rhis," for nose, and "itis," for inflammation. Put it all together and you've got "seasonal allergic nose inflammation." Whatever you call it, seasonal allergic rhinitis affects as many as 35 million Americans.

Here's what happens when you have hay fever. When an allergen (in this case, pollen) enters your body, your immune system mistakes it for a harmful intruder. It reacts by releasing powerful chemicals from mast cells and basophils. These chemicals (histamine is the best known) recruit other cells, which can remove the allergen and, through the process of inflammation, damage body tissue in the area.

With hay fever, the nose is the focus of the fray. That's because the allergens enter your body through the nostrils. Pollens are extremely small; the average pollen cell is about 50 microns long, less than the width of a human hair. On their way in, some pollens get stuck in your nose and release their proteins, which catch the attention of mast cells in the nose lining. Within as little as an hour, the mast cells go to work and symptoms appear.

The classic hay fever symptoms include sneezing, runny nose, itchy and watery eyes, and nasal congestion. But there are lots more. Here's a sample of things you may encounter:

- *The allergic "salute."* When your nose starts to drip, you instinctively rub your nostrils with the palm of your hand. This upward motion is called the allergic salute. Some children "salute" so often that they actually get a crease in the nose.
- *Allergic "shiners."* These are dark circles under the eyes caused by constant inflammation of the sinuses and nose lining.
- *Allergic conjunctivitis.* When pollen, dander, or other allergens touch the membranes around your eyelids, they may cause swelling, excessive watering, and itching. This condition is very common in people with hay fever. As many as 30 to 40 percent of people with seasonal allergies may also get conjunctivitis.

WHAT'S BOTHERING

Pollen comes from trees, grasses, and weeds. Depending on where you live, the pollen season can start as early as January and last into the

Region	Jan	Feb	Mar	Apr	May
Northeast CT, ME, MA, NH, RI, VT			Trees	Trees	Trees / Grass
Mid-Atlantic NJ, NY, PA, DE, MD, WV, DC			Trees	Trees	Trees / Grass
Southeast AL, AR, FL, GA, KY, LA, MS, NC, SC, TN, VA		Trees	Trees	Trees	Trees / Grass
Midwest IL, IN, IA, KS, MO, MN, OH, MI, NE, WI			Trees	Trees	Grass
Northeast WA, OR			Trees	Trees	Trees / Grass
Southwest AZ, OK, NV, NM, TX		Trees	Trees	Trees	Grass
Rocky Mountains CO, ID, MT, ND, SD, UT, WY					Trees
California South of San Francisco	Trees	Trees	Grass	Grass	Grass
California North of San Francisco	Trees	Trees	Trees	Trees / Grass	Trees / Grass

Trees   Grass

YOU NOW?

fall. This chart shows peak times for various types of pollen in all parts of the continental United States.

Jun	Jul	Aug	Sep	Oct	Nov	Dec

Source: American Academy of Allergy, Asthma and Immunology

Weeds

- *Loss of sense of smell and taste.* It's hard to smell or taste anything with a constantly stuffy nose.
- *Frequent nosebleeds.* The irritation of the delicate membrane lining the nose can cause it to bleed—usually a little, but sometimes a lot.
- *Frequent sinus infections.* These are caused by the constant swelling in the nose. When the nasal membranes are swollen, they don't drain the way they should. This keeps the nose from getting rid of bacteria, which can cause infections.
- *Delayed reactions.* In some people, a second set of symptoms can occur up to 24 hours after exposure to pollen. These include sneezing, itching, and dripping from the nose, eyes, and throat.

When it comes to seasonal allergies, ragweed grabs most of the spotlight in the eastern United States. And it certainly deserves the attention. About three in four people with allergic rhinitis are sensitive to ragweed pollen. But that late-summer bummer is only a small part of the allergy story. There's also tree and grass pollen to consider. Dozens of trees, shrubs, and grasses can cause allergic reactions. The American Academy of Allergy, Asthma, and Immunology estimates that as many as 40 percent of people with hay fever are sensitive to grass pollen and about 9 percent are sensitive to tree pollen. About one in four people with hay fever is sensitive to both grass and weed pollen—and a very unlucky 3 percent of folks with hay fever are allergic to all three types!

Depending on where you live and what you're allergic to, your allergies could last for months at a time. Trees can start pollinating as early as January in warm climates, followed within a month or two by flowering grasses. So by the time ragweed reaches its peak around Labor Day, you may already have suffered through nearly three seasons of sneezing.

The chart on pages 20-21 shows common trouble times for tree, grass, and weed allergies in different parts of the United States.

PERENNIAL PROBLEMS

If allergic rhinitis bothered you for only a few weeks each year, it might not be so bad. In between all the sniffles and sneezes, you could tell yourself that everything will pass when the pollen peters out. But for many people, airborne allergens are a problem all year long. That's because it's not just pollen that's causing the problem. Several other common substances can cause allergic reactions, too—and can last all year long. That's why they fall into the category of perennial allergic rhinitis.

Here are some of the most common perennial pests.

Dust. When's the last time you cleaned behind the bookcase in the den? Chances are, there's a dust bunny or two lurking in your house somewhere. And it's full of stuff that can cause allergic reactions.

The biggest problem with dust is the mites that contribute to it. Mites (the most common of which is *Dermatophagoides pteronyssinus*) are tiny creatures that belong to the arachnid family, along with spiders, ticks, and chiggers. Mites live in bedding and upholstered furniture, and their body parts and waste make up a portion of dust. Under a microscope, mites look like hump-backed, saw-toothed, eight-legged monsters capable of eating humans for Sunday brunch.

ALLERGY LOOK-ALIKES

If it looks like an allergy and feels like an allergy, it usually is an allergy. But not always. Sometimes people develop symptoms that mimic allergic reactions yet are caused by other factors. These problems are called **nonallergic rhinitis**.

Doctors have identified a number of different causes for nonallergic rhinitis. Here are a few of the most important ones.

Vasomotor rhinitis. Also called irritant rhinitis, it may be triggered by strong fumes, weather changes, emotional stress, or other factors. No one is quite sure how or why this problem occurs, but it seems to be more common in adults than in children.

Structural rhinitis. Sometimes the way your nose is built can cause problems. There's a wall of cartilage between your nostrils called the septum. If this is out of place, because it either grew that way or was injured, it can cause chronic inflammation in the nose. The only way to fix this is surgery.

Eosinophilic rhinitis. Eosinophils are blood cells that are part of the immune system. Like basophils and mast cells, they are capable of releasing chemicals to fight off intruders—especially parasites like worms. While eosinophils play a role in allergic reactions, they are often associated with nonallergic rhinitis.

Neutrophilic rhinosinusitis. Neutrophils are another type of blood cell. They are also called phagocytes. Their job is to devour and destroy harmful substances in the body. While they go about their business, they can cause nasal congestion and other symptoms that are similar to those of allergies. This type of rhinitis is usually caused by an infection in the sinuses.

Infectious rhinitis. This is a fancy name for the common cold and flu. To fight off the viruses that cause these illnesses, your body reacts by creating inflammation in the nose. This results in a runny nose, congestion, sneezing, and watery eyes.

How can you tell the difference between all the different types of rhinitis? Well, it can get a little complicated sometimes. Here are some basic guidelines.

- **Seasonal allergic rhinitis:** Caused by pollen or molds. Lasts as long as the airborne allergen is present. Symptoms include runny nose, congestion, watery or itchy eyes, and sneezing. No fever or muscle aches.
- **Perennial allergic rhinitis:** Caused by dust, dander, and indoor mold. Can last year-round, depending on the presence of allergens. Symptoms are the same as for seasonal allergic rhinitis, but often occur when no pollen is present, such as in the cold of winter.
- **Nonallergic rhinitis:** Aggravated primarily by fumes and changes in weather. Will last as long as the substance that causes symptoms is present. Symptoms are similar to those of allergic rhinitis, but usually there are less itching and sneezing and no eye symptoms. Can be difficult to pinpoint; you may need to consult an allergist.
- **Infectious rhinitis:** Caused by viruses or bacteria. Usually lasts 7 to 10 days, then disappears. Symptoms are similar to those of allergic rhinitis, but also can include fever and muscle aches.

It may not seem terribly important to identify the source of your nose woes. After all, congestion is congestion. But treatments can be quite different. What may seem like a persistent cold may actually be an allergic reaction. No amount of cough syrup or aspirin is going to make it go away. Rather, the best way to handle allergies is to avoid the allergen or to take antihistamines and other allergy medications. If you have nonallergic rhinitis, on the other hand, allergy medications won't be much help, and you'll have to figure out what's causing the problem so you can learn to avoid it.

In a very real (and somewhat disgusting) sense, that's exactly what they do. Dust mites live by eating the flakes of skin that people and other animals shed from their bodies every day. This is a useful job, actually; without mites, we could be up to our ears in old skin. And it's not the mites themselves that cause allergic reactions in people, anyway. It's their waste products. After they digest their meals, mites excrete proteins that we sometimes breathe. About 1 in 10 people appears to be sensitive to dust mite excretions. Nearly 80 percent of children with asthma are affected by them.

The average house contains millions and millions of dust mites (the highest known concentration of mites was 18,875 in one gram of dust). Each mite creates 10 to 20 waste particles each day, and individual mites live for about a month. You'll find mites just about everywhere people lounge or sleep—on mattresses, sofas, carpets, car seats, and even clothes.

Mold. Any house that has dark and warm places probably has mold. As with dust mites, it's not the mold itself that causes allergic reactions. It's the spores that mold creates in order to reproduce. When mold releases its spores, the spores float throughout the house, helped along by air vents, fans, and leaky vacuum cleaners. When we breathe in the spores, our immune systems go on the defensive, causing the classic allergy symptoms.

Pet dander. Proteins from your pet's shed skin are common household allergy triggers. Pet saliva (especially from cats) also may cause problems, despite what you may have heard about how clean a pet's tongue is supposed to be.

TAKING ALLERGIES SERIOUSLY

Everybody knows at least one tough guy. He's the fellow who shows up at work with a 103-degree fever. He claims he's never taken an aspirin in his life. And he says that he'd rather let his illness "run its course" than take action to stop it.

Well, that kind of bravado can get you in hot water with allergies. Ignoring seasonal or perennial allergic rhinitis can cause additional problems that may be harder to fix. Here are a few.

Sinus infections. The medical term is sinusitis. Sinuses are hollow cavities located behind your nose. They contain mucus, which naturally flows down your nostrils and out your nose.

Mucus contains a lot of bacteria. Your sinuses can usually handle the bacteria because they ship it, along with the mucus, out of your body. But when your nose swells up, bacteria can get trapped in your sinuses, where it may multiply and cause a nasty infection. The result is acute sinus pain, headaches, and difficulty breathing. The National Institutes of Health estimates that 32 million Americans suffer from chronic sinusitis, which can last for weeks, months, or even years if left untreated.

Many things can cause sinusitis. Colds and the flu are often a problem, since they can swell your nasal passages shut. But the single biggest cause of sinusitis is allergic rhinitis, either from seasonal problems like ragweed or from perennial problems like dust.

Getting rid of sinusitis can be tricky. First, you'll need to take antibiotics. These help your body kill off the bacteria. Second, you'll have to make sure that your sinuses remain open, which is why your doctor may recommend that you take a decongestant and maybe an antihistamine or an inhaled steroid. Finally, you'll have to deal with the underlying cause of the infection—the blockages in the nose. If these are caused by allergies, you're going to have to learn to avoid the allergens that cause reactions. We talk more about controlling your exposure to allergens in chapter 9.

Nasal polyps. The constant swelling of your nasal passages can trigger the growth of benign little sacs called polyps on the inside of your nose. When polyps get large enough, you may have difficulty breathing through one or both nostrils. Nearly 30 percent of adults with nonallergic rhinitis will eventually develop polyps. There's no medication to treat polyps; the only way to get rid of them is to have them surgically removed.

Ear infections. Most children will get an ear infection or two without having long-term problems. But if these infections are allowed to persist, or if they happen too often, they can cause permanent damage to the ear. Allergic rhinitis appears to play a significant role in causing ear infections. Studies have found that as many as 35 percent of kids with chronic ear infections also have allergic rhinitis. The link between the two isn't clear at this point. Some experts believe that allergic reactions may block the eustachian tubes, which lead from the middle ear to the nasal passages, allowing infections to form inside.

Asthma. There's a very strong connection between asthma and allergic rhinitis. Nearly 6 in every 10 people with asthma also suffer from hay fever or perennial rhinitis. Many times, asthma attacks are triggered by the same allergens that cause allergic reactions. Asthma

POLYP PROBLEMS

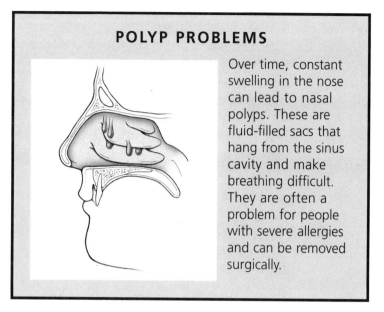

Over time, constant swelling in the nose can lead to nasal polyps. These are fluid-filled sacs that hang from the sinus cavity and make breathing difficult. They are often a problem for people with severe allergies and can be removed surgically.

is a serious condition. It affects more than 10 million Americans and can make breathing extremely difficult during attacks. In some cases, it can even be fatal. Needless to say, people with allergic rhinitis and asthma must work extra hard to avoid allergens.

Social and psychological problems. Allergic rhinitis can be hard on more than just your body. Leading allergy researchers believe that it can lead to additional problems like frustration, embarrassment, irritability, and poor sleep. For children, things can be even harder. Many kids with uncontrolled allergies find it hard to get interested in school and social activities. This can lead to absenteeism from school and may even lead to temper tantrums and other behavioral problems. Some studies have shown links between allergic rhinitis and shyness and depression, too.

FIGHTING BACK

With all this at stake, you can see why it makes so much sense to get your allergies under control. It's more than just the inconvenience of sneezing and blowing your nose constantly. It's about keeping yourself healthier and happier for years to come.

In the battle against allergic rhinitis, you have three key weapons. The first is avoidance. If you don't breathe in pollen, you won't get hay fever. Of course, that's easier said than done. In reality, the best you can hope for is to limit your exposure. The same goes for perennial problems like dust and dander. You can dust your house 14 times a day and still not get rid of all the mites. But you can employ some strategies to keep things under control. We talk about these in more detail in chapter 9.

The second strategy against allergies is to treat the symptoms. When you find yourself wheezing and sneezing, it just doesn't make sense to tough it out. Between over-the-counter and prescription medicines, there are plenty of treatments that will keep your symptoms in check.

We'll discuss the different types, brands, and dosages of allergy medicines in more detail in chapter 10, but here's a quick summary.

Antihistamines. These are the best drugs for stopping sneezing and itching. They work by blocking the effects of histamine—one of the chemicals released from mast cells and basophils during an allergic reaction. The biggest problem with antihistamines is that many of them are sedating; they cause some people to feel drowsy and can be dangerous to take if you need to drive a vehicle. Fortunately, there are newer antihistamines that do not produce drowsiness, although they are available only by prescription. The other problem with antihistamines is that they're most effective when you take them before exposure to allergens. You can't wait until symptoms begin. You'll have to learn to anticipate when you're going to breathe in pollen. Once an intense allergic reaction starts, antihistamines are of limited use.

Decongestants. These medicines work quickly to dry up secretions and reduce the swelling inside your nose, making it easier to breathe. Decongestants are available as pills and sprays in both over-the-counter and prescription formulas. Many drug makers have combined antihistamines and decongestants in one pill, which you may find convenient. The only major problem with decongestant sprays is something called the rebound effect. If you use nasal sprays too often to fight congestion, you may end up causing more congestion instead. So you'll have to be careful.

Corticosteroids. These are the strongest of the antiallergy medicines. They're available only by prescription as nasal sprays, pills, and injections. Corticosteroids are highly effective at relieving symptoms and at stopping allergic reactions before they start. When taken properly, they're also quite safe—especially the nasal spray.

If you can't avoid allergens, and medications don't give you the relief you seek, there's one final choice: immunotherapy. These are also called allergy shots. Over the course of weeks, months, or even years, you'll receive injections that contain tiny amounts of the allergen or allergens that you react to. In time, your body will build up a tolerance to the allergen, reducing or eliminating your reactions. If this sounds too good to be true, well, sometimes it is. It can take a long, long time to be effective. It doesn't always work. And you'll need to take booster shots to keep up your "immunity" to the allergen. Still, if there's no other way to deal with your allergies, immunotherapy may be your best bet. For more information on allergy shots, see chapter 11.

HINTS TO HALT HAY FEVER

Every year, come hay fever season, you probably ask yourself the same two questions: (1) "What did I do to deserve this? and (2) "Where can I go to get away from it?" Unfortunately, the answers are (1) nothing and (2) nowhere. Allergies just happen in some people—and there's simply no running from ragweed.

There are about 35 species of ragweed, which belongs to the botanical family *Ambrosia*. Such a sweet name for such a nasty weed! Ragweed plants can grow as high as five feet. Once they mature in mid- to late summer, the flowers release their dreaded pollen until the plants are killed by frost.

Ragweed grows almost everywhere in the continental United States. There are precious few places (far-southern Florida and far-northern Maine, for example) that don't have it. Even Hawaii and Alaska have some ragweed. Moving from the country to the city won't usually work, either. That's because pollen is so light that it can travel for miles before landing in your nose.

Besides, ragweed is just one source of allergy-causing pollens. There are so many different kinds of grasses and trees and weeds that you're likely to run into something that makes you sneeze no matter where you go.

You simply can't escape pollen. But you can learn to hide from it when it's at its worst. Pollen will only cause problems if you breathe it into your nose and throat. So lying low in an air-conditioned environment during high-pollen periods can really help.

The first thing you need to do is figure out what general types of pollen make you sneeze. For this, a little detective work will help. What times of the year are your allergies at their worst? Spring? Summer? Fall? Knowing this will help you narrow the field. For example, if you feel fine during the spring and early summer, then you're probably not allergic to pollen from trees like elms, birches, poplars, sycamores, maples, walnuts, or cypress.

On the other hand, if you start sneezing in the late spring and early summer, grasses may be the problem. These include Bermuda grass, timothy, sweet vernal, rye, and some varieties of bluegrass, to name a few. And if your symptoms don't start until later in the summer, it's probably ragweed, some other weed, or an outdoor mold.

Identifying exactly which pollens cause you trouble isn't always the most important thing. That's because trees, grasses, and weeds bloom at predictable times every year. If you know that you're allergic to some type of tree pollen, you can be sure that it will be present every spring—but not in the fall. You'll only have to be on high allergy alert during your worst season.

However, if you and your doctor decide that immunotherapy is an attractive option, you'll need to pinpoint the pollen source. Allergy shots are very specific; getting a shot against ragweed isn't going to help you against birch pollen. For this kind of accuracy, you'll probably need to take some skin or blood tests. We discuss these tests in chapter 8.

What if you have hay fever symptoms in the winter months? Well, if you live in a warm climate, your allergies may be caused by pollen even in December. If not, you may discover that pollen isn't really your problem after all. Instead, you could have perennial allergic rhinitis—caused by dust, indoor mold, or pet dander. If you suspect this is the problem, talk to your doctor. It may be a good idea to get some skin tests to determine exactly what you're allergic to. Once you figure that out, turn to chapter 9 for lots of tips on controlling allergens within your home and surroundings.

Short of sealing your doors and windows with plastic and waiting for winter, there's no way to completely avoid pollen. But here are a few tips that can help limit your exposure.

Know the score. Even at the peak of allergy season, some days are worse than others. That's why it's not a bad idea to check the local pollen count. Many organizations and weather services count the number of pollen cells in the air each day, then compile and release reports for newspapers and television and radio stations.

Here's how it works. Technicians attach an adhesive material to a rod, which is placed on a rooftop and hooked up to a rotating arm. The rod spins around, catching pollen on the adhesive. After a period of time, the rod is removed and the adhesive is placed in a dye. This dye makes it easier to count the number of pollen granules. The technician then counts the granules under a microscope. This figure is the pollen count and is expressed as the number of grains per cubic meter of air.

A pollen count of 100 or fewer grains is considered low. Anything between 100 and 500 grains is considered moderate. Readings between 500 and 1,000 are termed high, and anything over 1,000 grains is considered very high. Similar readings for the amount of mold spores in the air are also tabulated.

What does this mean for you? Well, consider the low reading as a green light. If you have work to do outside, this is a good time to get going. The moderate reading is like a yellow light. You can expect to feel some symptoms unless you take antihistamines prior to venturing outside. A high reading is a red light. Go outside at your peril! A very high count is like a red light flashing at a railroad intersection, and you can hear the locomotive's whistle. Stay indoors! Keep the windows shut. If you need to cool things down in your car or home, use the air conditioner; it can be set to recirculate inside air only.

Unfortunately, pollen counts are not perfect. For one thing, they're taken the day before they're released to the public. So you won't be sure what today's pollen count is until tomorrow. That's of little use if pollen picks up overnight. Still, it's probably the best system around right now. If you have access to the Internet, you can find a daily pollen and spore count from the National Allergy Bureau. The bureau is run by the American Academy of Allergy, Asthma, and Immunology. You can find its maps at *http://weather.yahoo.com/graphics/pollen/*.

Don't get winded. Even without a pollen count, you can tell when some days are going to be tougher than others. One of the biggest factors is wind. When it's whipping, you can bet that it's carrying a mother lode of pollen and mold. But when it's calm, the pollen settles and causes less trouble. Warm, dry air tends to keep pollen counts high, but rainy, cool weather can sometimes beat the pollen to the ground.

Generally speaking, early morning is the best time to get things done outside. Airborne pollen is usually at its lowest between 5 a.m. and 10 a.m. This is a good time to cut the grass, go for a bike ride, or walk the dogs. During peak pollen periods, consider wearing a pollen-filtering face mask to keep the grains away from the inside of your nose. If you must go outside when you think pollen counts are high, try taking an anti-histamine 30 minutes to an hour before you leave the house. This can help thwart symptoms before they start.

Run for the beach. Although you'll encounter pollen and mold almost everywhere you go, there's one place that is better than any other: the seaside. Ragweed doesn't grow well in areas along the northern Atlantic coast. Plus, the prevailing daytime wind comes off the water, so there's not likely to be as much pollen in the air. That doesn't mean you should leave your medicines at home, however, since you can encounter some pollen and mold just about everywhere during peak seasons.

Ban cantaloupe. Some common foods have proteins similar to those found in pollens and molds. Eating these foods during peak hay fever season can make allergic reactions worse. If you're allergic to ragweed, for example, watermelon, cantaloupes, and honeydews may cause extra problems in the mouth and throat. The herb chamomile may cause you problems, too.

There are dozens of these possible interactions. Until you know exactly what you're allergic to, there's no sense worrying about food-related cross-reactions. Once your doctor identifies your allergens, he will let you know which foods could cause you trouble.

Incidentally, insecticides that contain pyrethrum also can cause hay fever symptoms. That's because the chemical is made from chrysanthemums—a flower that's closely related to ragweed!

Now, we're going to look more closely at one of the most serious of all allergy-related conditions: asthma. Why only a portion of people with allergies get asthma isn't clearly understood. But one thing is certain: Learning how to deal with the causes can improve your lifestyle dramatically.

CHAPTER 3

Asthma: Lessons for Your Lungs

We know a lot less about asthma than we'd like to. After decades of research, doctors still don't know the cause. And after years of testing, there's still no cure.

But there's one thing experts are certain about: Almost every one of the 14 million Americans with asthma can keep it under control. That means:

- No frequent symptoms of wheezing, coughing, shortness of breath, or tightness in the chest
- Sleeping through the night without symptoms
- No missed school or work due to asthma
- No emergency room visits or stays in the hospital
- Few, if any, side effects from asthma medication
- Full participation in physical activities

All this may sound too good to be true. But believe us, it's possible. You (or your child) can lead a normal, active life with asthma—as long as you're willing to work at it. Notice that the key is *you*. You'll have to take your medication. You'll have to monitor your lung capacity. You'll have to learn to avoid your asthma triggers. And you'll have to know when it's time to back off a little to keep your asthma under control.

In a bit, we'll explain common strategies for dealing with asthma—everything from dusting your bedroom to using an emergency inhaler. But first, let's take a look at what asthma is and what it does.

THE BREATH ROBBER

Asthma is a respiratory disease that affects the lungs. It is **chronic,** meaning that it lasts a long time—sometimes all your life. And it is **episodic,** meaning that sometimes you'll have severe symptoms that make it very difficult to breathe.

To explain asthma, we have to start with your lungs. These are magnificent organs that take oxygen from the air and deliver it to your bloodstream. All the cells in your body need oxygen to survive. Without it, your brain, heart, liver, and other organs couldn't function—and neither could you.

When you breathe in, air passes through your nose and mouth and down the windpipe (the **trachea**). At its bottom, the trachea splits into two parts, called **bronchi.** The bronchi, in turn, divide into smaller passageways that feed air to pockets in the lungs called lobes. Each lung has five lobes. Inside these lobes are extremely small passageways called **bronchioles.** And at the end of each bronchiole are air sacs called **alveoli.** Tiny blood vessels called capillaries are attached to the alveoli. Their job is to take the oxygen from the alveoli and carry it into the bloodstream. At the same time, the capillaries drop off carbon dioxide, a waste product that's a normal part of cell metabolism. When you exhale, the carbon dioxide follows the exact opposite path as the oxygen: from the alveoli to the bronchioles to the bronchi and out the trachea.

Your lungs are very good at their job. We breathe every minute of every day, whether we're sprinting down a soccer field or are fast asleep in bed. It's something most of us take for granted—until something blocks the flow of air, like a cold, allergies, bronchitis, pneumonia, or asthma.

As we've seen, no one is really sure what causes asthma. But we do know that certain things can trigger periodic asthma attacks—including allergens like dust, pollen, pet dander, air pollution, cigarette or wood smoke, strong fumes, and even changing weather or cold air. When an asthma attack strikes, three things happen in the lungs.

1. **Inflammation.** The insides of the bronchioles swell, narrowing the passageways. This makes it harder for air to move in and out of the lungs.

2. **Constriction.** The muscles wrapped around the bronchioles tighten, which further narrows the openings.

3. **Mucus production.** Mucus is a cleaning agent in the lungs that helps wash out foreign particles. But during an asthma attack, excess mucus gets released. This takes up space in the passageways that carry air, making it even harder to breathe.

The result of all this is the classic asthma symptoms: wheezing, gasping for breath, coughing, and a feeling of tightness in the chest. Asthma episodes can last for hours or even days, depending on how well you treat them with your medication.

Asthma usually begins in childhood, although adult-onset cases also occur. Asthma rates vary widely around the world, but in the United States about 7 percent to 10 percent of all children have asthma to some degree. This makes it the most widespread chronic disease among American children. Many times, the symptoms will become less serious as the child ages. In fact, the symptoms disappear altogether in about 50 percent of the cases as children reach adulthood.

Unfortunately, asthma is on the rise. In 1980, about 7 million Americans had asthma. But that number had doubled by 1994. Some experts believe that bad indoor air quality and increased exposure to allergic "triggers" could be causing the rise, but no one knows for sure. And the numbers may be even worse than we suspect. Asthma remains the most underdiagnosed and under-treated chronic disease in this country.

Although asthma is very treatable, it can be danger-ous if you don't keep it under control. Despite better medicines and a better understanding of how asthma works, people with asthma, as a group, go to the hospital nearly half a million times a year. They have more than 100 million days of restricted activity. More than 5,000 people in the United States die of asthma every year.

Anyone can develop asthma. But certain people have a higher risk than others. The disease is frequently asso-ciated with allergies. That means that "atopic" people—those who tend to produce high amounts of antibodies to allergens like dust, pollen, mold, and other sub-stances—are more apt to have asthma. There's a genetic link, so asthma seems to run in families. But just because you have allergies or asthma doesn't necessarily mean your children will have them, too. It's sort of a hit-or-miss proposition, and no one is quite sure why.

In adults who get asthma, allergies don't seem to play a role as much as in children. However, conditions like sinusitis and nasal polyps do seem to be involved. In addition, some adults get "occupational" asthma, which is caused by exposure to chemicals in the workplace. This may account for as much as 5 percent to 10 percent of asthma cases in America—and even more in other countries, such as Japan. Because adult-onset and occupational asthma aren't related to allergies, we're not going to talk too much about them in this chapter. But much of the advice that follows will be of use to people who suffer from these forms of the disease, too.

Asthma comes in degrees. Some people have only occasional, short-lived episodes, whereas others have symptoms that occur almost all the time. The National Institutes of Health has divided people with asthma into four categories called steps.

Step 1: Mild Intermittent. This is the least severe type of asthma. People with Step 1 asthma have symptoms no more than two times a week and nighttime symptoms no more than two times a month. In between asthma episodes, they have no symptoms at all. Episodes can last from a few hours to a few days, and lung capacity is no worse than 80 percent of normal. (We'll talk about measuring lung capacity in just a bit.)

Step 2: Mild Persistent. People with Step 2 asthma have symptoms more than twice a week but never more than once a day. They also have nighttime symptoms more than twice a week. The episodes are often severe enough to restrict physical activity, but their lung function still isn't worse than 80 percent of normal during asthma episodes.

Step 3: Moderate Persistent. People with Step 3 asthma have symptoms every day and nighttime symptoms more than once a week. They usually use an inhaler every day to control their asthma. They have episodes more than twice a week, and the episodes may last for days. Their physical activity is restricted during episodes, when their lung capacity is between 61 percent and 80 percent.

Step 4: Severe Persistent. People at this level have continual symptoms during the day, frequent nighttime symptoms, and frequent episodes. Their physical activity is limited. During episodes, their lung capacity is 60 percent of normal or less.

How you treat asthma largely depends on which category you fall into. For example, people with Step 1 asthma don't need regular daily medication, but people with Step 4 asthma may need high doses of corticosteroids to keep their asthma in check.

Every stage of asthma requires a doctor's supervision, of course. The ultimate goal is to become as independent as possible, but this is not a disease that you should try to handle on your own. Effective asthma management is a partnership between you and your doctor. Working with your physician, you can learn the triggers for your asthma, how to self-monitor your symptoms, and when to call for help. You can learn to keep what is called a "peak flow" diary to keep track of your progress. And you can learn when to give yourself special rescue medicines.

The tips that follow are meant only as a supplement to your doctor's care and advice.

There are three main ways to deal with asthma. First, you can work to prevent asthma attacks by learning what causes your episodes. In many cases, simple lifestyle changes—and better housecleaning—can make life much easier for you or your child. Or you can take medications, both to prevent asthma attacks and to deal with them once they start. Finally, there's immunotherapy, which can make your body much less sensitive to asthma triggers. It's not for everyone, but sometimes it can be a real blessing. Since many people can control asthma the easy way—with lifestyle changes—let's discuss this first.

STOPPING THE SOURCE

For some people, it's the family cat. For others, it's ragweed. And for lots of people with asthma, it's hard to tell. We're talking about triggers—the allergens or irritants that can cause asthma attacks.

As we've seen, asthma is often linked to allergies. So the same allergens that cause some people to sneeze or get a stuffy nose can trigger attacks in people with asthma. Here are the main allergic triggers.

House dust mites. No matter how clean your house is, you probably have millions of these microscopic mites. They're on your pillows, your furniture, your bedding, your carpet, and your clothes. They excrete a protein that's a very potent asthma trigger.

Molds. Mold lives where it's dark and damp. That means showers, bathrooms, basements, rotting leaves, firewood, and many other places. Mold reproduces by creating spores that float through the air. Breathing in these spores can cause allergic reactions in many people.

ROACHES: THE HIDDEN TRIGGER

There's one additional allergen that causes problems for many people with asthma. It's not a pleasant topic, but here it is: cockroaches.

Salivary secretions, droppings, and disintegrated body parts from cockroaches are now believed to be allergens. They contain proteins that may cause allergic reactions and asthma episodes in people who are sensitive to them. And whether we like to think about it or not, cockroaches are very common. One Johns Hopkins study in Baltimore found that 81 percent of urban households in the city had cockroach allergens. The allergens were less common in rural areas but were still often present. Nationwide, cockroach allergens are believed to be present in about 23 percent of all households.

Some experts believe that cockroach allergens are one of the big reasons for the increase in asthma cases across the country, especially in inner-city areas. Children from poor urban families are far more likely to develop asthma than those from more affluent suburban or rural areas. One study found that 37 percent of inner-city children with asthma were sensitive to cockroach allergen. To put this in perspective, 35 percent were sensitive to dust mites and 23 percent were sensitive to cat dander.

How can you deal with this distasteful problem? Here are some suggestions:

- Use insect sprays or pesticide treatments. Make sure the person with asthma is not in the house when it's being sprayed or treated.
- Air out the house for several hours after spraying. Open windows and doors, and use fans to blow out the fumes.

- ◆ If pesticides don't solve the problem, place roach traps in the insect's favorite places: under sinks, behind refrigerators, and so on.
- ◆ Cover food and put it away in cabinets or your refrigerator. This includes pet food.
- ◆ Clean up crumbs, spills, or puddles of water or other liquids.
- ◆ Scrub grease from stove tops, ovens, counters, walls, and so on.
- ◆ Store garbage in closed containers.

Pollens. The most familiar pollen is ragweed. But many weeds, trees, and garden plants produce pollen that can lead to allergic reactions and asthma attacks.

Pet dander. Flakes of animal skin contain proteins that trigger allergies and asthma in many people.

Foods and medicines. In rare cases, allergies to food proteins can trigger an asthma episode. Foods containing preservatives called sulfites can sometimes be the culprit. Sulfites are often added to foods like dried fruit, beer, wine, processed potatoes, and shrimp.

Sensitivities to aspirin and related painkillers are more common. People with asthma who believe that these medicines may have made their condition worse should consult their doctors.

Controlling all of these triggers can be a time-consuming process. In some cases, it can be heartbreaking, too; more than a few people with asthma have had to say good-bye to a pet. But reducing your exposure to allergens can make all the difference in dealing with asthma. We talk much more about avoiding common allergens in chapter 9.

Not all asthma triggers are allergy related. Many common substances can cause asthma episodes even when they don't cause allergies. Here are some of the main ones.

Viral infections. Some asthma triggers come from within. For example, respiratory infections like head colds and the flu can cause episodes. The best remedy for this cause is to stay healthy. That means avoiding people with colds and washing your hands frequently, which will help wash away germs before they make you sick. If you have asthma, you should ask your doctor for an annual vaccine against the flu.

Tobacco smoke. Airborne particles from cigarettes, cigars, and pipes can get into the lungs of people with asthma and cause attacks. Don't ever smoke in the bedroom of a person with asthma. In fact, avoid smoking in the house entirely. If someone in the house is a smoker, have her smoke outside (and encourage her to quit!). Finally, avoid smoking areas in public. Make sure you sit in nonsmoking sections of airports and restaurants.

Wood smoke and kerosene smoke. Sure, these stoves can keep you warm, but they can be a nightmare for people with asthma. Don't use a woodstove unless it's tightly sealed. Open fireplaces are almost always a bad idea. If you use a kerosene space heater, vent it to the outside or switch to an electric model instead.

Aerosol sprays. The fine mist from spray cans can irritate the lungs of people with asthma. Try using products in liquid or solid form instead of a spray.

Strong odors. Anything from powerful perfume to paint stripper can trigger an asthma reaction. Keep the smells down!

Acid reflux. Doctors have found that when powerful stomach acids slip uphill into the esophagus, asthma attacks may occur. The best way to handle this problem is to avoid eating and drinking for at least three hours before going to bed. Or you can raise the head of your bed by six to eight inches, which will help keep stomach acids down where they belong. Medications that control heartburn can also help. Just be sure to talk to your doctor before taking any new medication.

Cold and dry air. This is another common trigger. If the air affects you, try to avoid strenuous physical activity when it's cold out or use a bronchodilating inhaler first. And wear a scarf that covers your nose and mouth. That will help warm up the air before it reaches your lungs.

Exercise. A strenuous workout can cause asthma attacks. This condition is known as exercise-induced asthma, and almost everyone with asthma has it to some degree. This condition doesn't have to stop a life of physical activity. In fact, many great athletes have overcome asthma.

Some activities are more likely to cause asthma attacks than others. These include distance running and strenuous bicycling. Many other activities are perfectly fine, including walking, jogging, leisure bicycling, and swimming. Swimming, in fact, may be especially good because pool areas are warm and humid. And exercising in a horizontal position may help clear mucus from the lungs, too.

In many cases, people with exercise-induced asthma need to take medications before they begin exercising. It's also a good idea to warm up before exercising, which helps relieve chest tightness. Doctors recommend stretching and breaking a sweat about 30 minutes prior to beginning strenuous exercise. And don't exercise when you have a viral infection, when pollen counts are high, or when the weather is especially hot or cold.

ASTHMA MEDICINES

Even people with mild intermittent asthma will need to take medication occasionally. Others will need to use medications every day, sometimes several times a day. Treating asthma with medication is a very individualized process. Two people with asthma will invariably use different medications, doses, and frequency to control their symptoms. So there's no such thing as an "ideal" treatment plan.

There are two main classes of asthma medication, those for quick relief and those for long-term control. The quick-relief medicines are known as **short-acting beta$_2$-adrenergic agonists**. These are often used to help people who have just started having an asthma attack. They work like the body's own adrenaline hormone, but are designed to relax the lungs without affecting the heart or blood pressure. They can be taken in tablet form, by injection, or—most commonly—through an inhaler.

Here are three common short-acting drugs used in inhalers.

- Albuterol (brand names Proventil, Ventolin)
- Metaproterenol (brand names Alupent, Metaprel)
- Terbutaline (brand name Brethaire)

These drugs work quickly, which is why they're often used as emergency or "rescue" inhalers when an asthma attack is beginning. They usually start to work within 1 to 15 minutes and can provide relief for 4 to 6 hours.

While most people use adrenergic drugs in the inhaler form, some people take pills instead. These can be used by young children who can't use an inhaler properly or by people who for some reason don't like or don't respond well to the inhaler.

Inhalers are easy to use, but there are a few steps that are important to follow.

- Take the medicine standing up.
- Shake the inhaler for a couple of seconds before using it.
- Hold the inhaler so the canister portion is higher than the mouthpiece.
- Hold the mouthpiece about an inch from your mouth, and open your mouth wide.
- Begin to inhale, then activate the canister to release the medication.
- Keeping your mouth open, continue to inhale until you have taken a full breath.
- Hold your breath for at least 10 seconds before exhaling.

Some people need more than one dose. Your doctor will let you know if you do.

When you first get an inhaler, it's a good idea to practice using it. When you're having an actual asthma attack, you don't want to be worrying about how to use the inhaler.

The drugs used in inhalers are very safe, but they may cause side effects in some people. These include nervousness, headaches, shakiness, rapid or pounding

THE BREATH CHECK

Take a deep breath. How do your lungs feel? Pretty good? OK? Lousy?

These aren't very objective standards. Even if you've had asthma for a long time, it's difficult to know just how well your lungs are functioning at different times. This can be a problem because having an accurate sense of lung function is essential for preventing asthma flare-ups. You need a tool that lets you know when an attack may be on the horizon so that you can take steps to avoid it. For many people, that tool is the peak flow meter.

The meter looks a little like a kazoo with a thermometer attached to one end. It measures how fast and hard you can blow air out of your lungs. When your lungs are working well, it can provide a baseline measurement. Once you know this number, you'll be able to tell when your lungs are a little off their game. This can be a warning signal to take some medication or ease up on the exercise—or even to see your doctor.

Your doctor will tell you whether you need a peak flow meter and exactly how to use it. But here's a quick review.

First, take measurements when your lungs are working well. Follow the instructions for using the peak flow meter (see box, page 55). Do the exercise three times and check the meter reading each time. Then take an average of the readings; this number is your baseline. Not everyone's baseline number is the same, so there's no point comparing. This is just a measurement of how much air you can exhale under normal conditions.

From now on, take at least two sets of readings a day—once after you wake up and once in the evening.

Do this before you take any asthma medication. Every time, take three readings and use the best of them. Then compare the result to your baseline. If it's between 80 percent and 100 percent of your baseline, you've got a green light to go ahead with normal activities. If it's between 50 percent and 80 percent, you're in the yellow zone—it's time to slow down a little because your lungs are not working at their best. If your doctor has given you a "rescue" inhaler to take when asthma attacks begin, this is the time to use it. Relax for a few minutes after using the medication, then take another meter reading. Once you're back above 80 percent of capacity, you're ready to resume your normal activities.

heartbeat, or nausea. If you have problems with side effects, talk with your doctor. Changing medications or dosages will often clear things up.

When you're trying to prevent asthma attacks, the best defense is a long-term medication. There are several types.

One is called **theophylline**. Actually, this medicine can be used either to prevent asthma episodes or to treat mild flare-ups. It is available in liquid, tablet, and capsule forms. Theophylline takes longer to work than inhalers, but the relief can last up to 24 hours. Theophylline comes in many brand names, including Elixophyllin, Slo-bid, Slo-phyllin, Somophyllin, Theo-Dur, Theolair, and Unidur.

Theophylline medications may cause undesirable side effects. These include abdominal pain, nausea, vomiting, headache, nervousness, loss of appetite, and insomnia. Theophylline medicines are available in slow-release formulations that may help smooth out the dosage levels and allow a person to take it only once or twice per day.

Asthma isn't caused only by a tightening of the air passages in the lungs. There's almost always swelling as well. This is why people with asthma often treat their symptoms with an anti-inflammatory drug.

A very helpful anti-inflammatory medication is **cromolyn sodium**. Cromolyn helps prevent the release of histamine and other chemicals that often occurs during an allergic reaction. This helps prevent swelling of bronchial passages in the lungs. It also can help prevent tightening of the airways due to exercise or breathing cold air.

Cromolyn isn't used to stop attacks. In fact, it may take as long as a month before it begins to work at all. Because its main job is prevention, it's usually taken by people who have frequent asthma episodes and need long-term help to control them. People often begin with theophylline for its quick action, then give it up once the cromolyn has started to work. It's a good swap because cromolyn has fewer potential side effects.

Cromolyn is an excellent drug for people who need to take medication every day. However, since it doesn't stop asthma attacks that are already underway, people using cromolyn often take other medications as well.

Users of cromolyn usually take it four times a day. There are three ways to take it. The first is with a nebulizer machine. This is the method most often used by young children. The second method is a metered-dose inhaler. It's not always as effective as the nebulizer in delivering the medicine, but it's a lot more convenient for patients who can follow instructions well. You can

THE PEAK FLOW METER

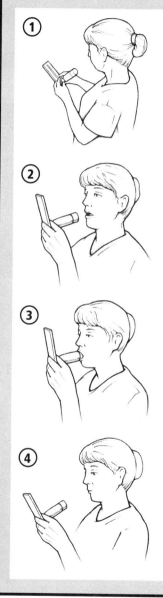

Using a peak flow meter can help a child or an adult with asthma tell when an attack may be approaching. Here's how to use it.

1. Set the meter to "0."

2. Stand up and take a deep breath.

3. Place the meter in your mouth and close your lips around it. Do not put your tongue in the hole. Blow out as hard and fast as you can.

4. Look at the reading. Write it down, then repeat twice more. The highest of the three readings will tell you how well your asthma is under control when compared to your base-line measurements.

carry it with you, and the doses are premeasured; one dose equals two puffs from the inhaler. Cromolyn is also taken in a powder form. The medicine is delivered into the lungs by a special machine called a spinhaler. This technique can be quite effective, although the powder may cause you to cough when you take it.

On the whole, cromolyn is free of serious side effects. About all you'll notice is an occasional wheeze and a bad taste in your mouth. You can take care of the bad taste by drinking a little water before and after taking the medicine.

One difficulty with using cromolyn is that your air passages need to be open before you take it. People using cromolyn often need to open up their airways with a puff inhaler first.

Nedocromil is another drug that acts pretty much the same way as cromolyn sodium. It also appears to be free of serious side effects.

Long-acting beta$_2$-agonists also are available. These come under the brand names Serevent, Volmax, and Proventil Repetabs. Unlike their short-acting cousins, these drugs can help prevent asthma symptoms in the dead of the night.

The most powerful anti-inflammatories are the **corticosteroids**, which reduce swelling and mucus production in the bronchioles. These are not the same drugs as the steroids used by bodybuilders.

Corticosteroids are extremely valuable because they can relieve severe cases of asthma that don't respond to other drugs. When adrenergic drugs or theophylline isn't working, using corticosteroids for a short time will often do the trick. Some people take corticosteroids on an ongoing basis, though this is only done as a last resort.

Corticosteroids are available in three forms: liquids, tablets, and inhalers. The oral forms are slower to work; it may take six or more hours before you start to get relief. But the oral medications are often stronger than the inhaled versions, so they're often the first choice— you may just have to wait a bit for the effects to kick in. The generic names for oral corticosteroids are prednisone, prednisolone, and methylprednisolone, and there are many different brands and generic forms. The inhaled steroids have the advantage of not producing the side effects caused by oral or injected steroids. They're available under the following names:

- Beclomethasone (brand names Beclovent, Vanceril)
- Flunisolide (brand name AeroBid)
- Triamcinolone (brand name Azmacort)
- Fluticasone (brand name Flovent)
- Budesonide (brand name Pulmicort)

Corticosteroids are usually used only when other types of drugs aren't working as well as they could. The problem with corticosteroids, especially the oral drugs, is side effects. If you take oral corticosteroids for only a couple of weeks at a time, the side effects may be minor: weight gain, increased appetite, stomach upset, and fluid retention. Taken long-term, however, oral corticosteroids may cause more serious problems, including retarded growth, weakened bones, high blood pressure, cataracts, muscle weakness and swelling, acne, excess body hair, and thinning of the skin.

That's a scary list. But people who can't control asthma any other way may have no choice but to risk the side effects.

Under no circumstances should anyone use long-term oral steroids until they (1) have exhausted all other drug options; (2) have made all possible efforts to control their exposure to allergens; and (3) have tried immunotherapy to ease their asthma symptoms if they are caused by allergies. Patients with sinus infections should not use long-term oral steroids until the infection has been treated because, in many cases, asthma will improve when the sinus infection disappears.

One last note for women: Many asthma drugs are safe to use during pregnancy. But it's very important to speak with your doctor if you're planning to have a child—and especially important if you're already pregnant. You may need to change medications or dosages. If you're taking allergy shots before you become pregnant, you'll probably be able to continue. But it's not a good idea to start the shots if you're already pregnant or plan to have a child soon.

Research has shown that women with asthma don't have a higher risk for problem pregnancies—if they control their condition. Women who don't control their asthma, however, are more likely to have low-birth-weight babies, possibly because the fetus does not receive enough oxygen from the mother when she is having asthma attacks.

Asthma will occasionally worsen late in pregnancy, but most women with asthma won't have problems during childbirth. In fact, they can often use the Lamaze breathing method during delivery despite having weaker lungs.

IMMUNOTHERAPY

Sometimes your best efforts to control asthma may come up a little short. Even if you vacuum all the dust, learn to exercise the correct way, and take the right medications in the right doses, you may still have asthma attacks. When this happens, you and your doctor may want to consider immunotherapy. It's appropriate only for about 1 person in 20, but when it works, it's very effective.

We'll talk more about immunotherapy in chapter 11, but here's a quick summary. Immunotherapy involves getting a series of injections that contain tiny amounts of the allergen you're allergic to. Each time you receive an injection, your body creates an antibody against that allergen. These antibodies intercept the allergens before they can trigger an asthma episode. Over time, you'll develop resistance to the allergen. In other words, you'll be less allergic than you were before.

Immunotherapy shots are given over the course of months or years because it will take a long time for you to build up resistance. Even then it may not be entirely successful. Immunotherapy works only when your doctor knows for sure that an allergen is causing your asthma—and he's able to identify exactly what the allergen is. In most cases, immunotherapy is only a last resort. It's always better to "treat" asthma by avoiding whatever it is that's taking your breath away.

The truth is, immunotherapy is not a miracle cure. It can be expensive. It usually requires booster shots many times a year, and it won't work when asthma is triggered by exercise, infections, smoke, fumes, cold air, or other problems. Even if you've had successful immunotherapy, you'll probably still need to take asthma medication and try to avoid whatever you're allergic to.

CHAPTER 4

Skin Allergies:
It's All in the Touch

Every Cub Scout and Brownie learned the rhyme:

> Leaflets three, let it be.
> Berries white, poisonous sight.

It's still good advice. If you've ever wandered off the beaten path without paying attention, you may have had your first brush—or your second or third—with poison ivy and then discovered just how miserable skin allergies can be.

So far we've been talking mostly about allergic reactions that start inside your body—in the stomach, intestines, lungs, and sinuses. Now we're going to look at allergies, like poison ivy, that are only skin deep. Many substances can cause your immune system to go bananas just by rubbing against your flesh. The results, needless to say, can be very irritating.

Unfortunately, skin allergies aren't limited to occasional nuisances like poison ivy. The National Institute for Occupational Safety and Health estimates that debilitating skin problems (including allergies) cause more than one-third of all job-related health problems in America. That's more than backaches, stress, carpal tunnel syndrome, or any other single workplace problem.

The good news is that you can save yourself from a whole rash of these rashes. The key is learning to identify—and then avoid—the substances that cause you grief. So let's get started on scratching skin allergies off your list of problems.

MAKING CONTACT

Most skin allergies are known collectively as contact dermatitis. As the name suggests, trouble starts when the outer layer of your skin (epidermis) touches (contacts) a foreign substance that causes a reaction. Not every case of contact dermatitis involves an allergic reaction. In fact, only about 1 in 10 cases is a true allergy. But allergic and nonallergic contact dermatitis may cause similar symptoms, so we'll talk about both of them in this chapter.

By now, you probably have memorized how most allergic reactions happen. A harmless allergen, usually a protein, enters the body and encounters the immune system. Specialized antibodies spot and grab on to the allergen. The immune system wrongly believes that the allergen is dangerous, so it releases strong chemicals from mast cells and basophils. These chemicals wipe out the allergen and in the process cause allergic symptoms.

Skin allergies are somewhat different. When the allergen comes in contact with skin, immune cells called T lymphocytes go to work. They release substances called lymphokines. One type of lymphokine sends out a call to cells known as macrophages. These are huge eating machines that destroy the allergen by engulfing and digesting it—along with human cells that contain traces of the allergen. Other lymphokines send signals that prevent the macrophages from leaving the scene until the job is done. Still others stimulate blood vessels at the site to pass extra fluid and inflammatory cells into nearby tissues. This swells and kills the cells, which the body has determined are "infected" by the harmless antigen.

The result is an unsightly mess. Skin allergies often cause swelling, redness, tenderness, and rashes. Fortunately, the allergic reaction is localized; that is, it doesn't go any farther than the area of skin that rubbed against the allergen in the first place. That's much different than other types of allergies, which can cause symptoms all over your body.

Allergic reactions on the skin usually take a while to show up. While you can start feeling a food allergy immediately, you're not likely to notice a poison ivy rash for 24 to 72 hours. It just takes a while longer for the T-cell gang to get going.

Most skin allergies are not life-threatening. Sure, you can get a nasty rash and terrible itching for a few days. But that's about as far as things go in most cases. The macrophages remove the dead cells, the skin heals—and you're no worse for the experience.

Skin allergies involve a process called sensitization. The first time you touch poison ivy, you won't get a rash. That's because your body has never seen the allergen before. The T cells take note of the intruder but don't attack it full force. The next time you touch poison ivy, however, you probably won't be so lucky. Once you've been sensitized, your T cells will react strongly every time they see the allergen. It usually takes about a week after your first exposure to the allergen before you become fully sensitized to it. In some cases, it takes several exposures before you get sensitized. But after that, it's time to break out the calamine lotion!

THE MAIN CAUSES

Just about anything that touches your skin is a potential allergen. But some substances are far more likely to cause a reaction than others. Here's a summary of the most common offenders.

Poison ivy/poison oak/poison sumac. Researchers believe that one-half to three-quarters of Americans are allergic to these nasty green plants. In truth, "the poisons" aren't really poisonous. But the oily resin that they produce, called urushiol, is an allergen. When you get the stuff on your skin, you're likely to pay the price—sometimes for days.

You must come in skin contact with the plant or its oils to get a rash. If you get a poison ivy rash but can't remember touching it, one of two things probably happened. You may have touched it two or three days earlier and only noticed when your skin broke out. Or the oil may have gotten onto work gloves, clothes, pet fur, shoes, hats, or work tools. When you touch them later—even months later—the oil can still be active and cause a reaction.

Poison ivy and poison oak each have three glossy-green leaflets. They can grow as a single plant or a vine. The leaves can vary greatly from plant to plant; some are smooth on the edges, whereas others are irregular.

LEAFLETS THREE...

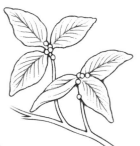

poison ivy

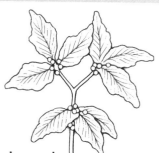

poison oak

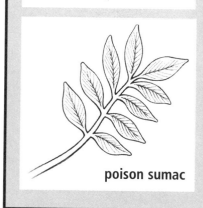

poison sumac

The only way to avoid poison ivy, poison oak, and poison sumac is to know what the plants look like. All three are native to North America and are found everywhere from wooded areas to backyard planters. They grow as clusters of climbing vines or as shrubby plants.

Poison ivy and **poison oak** are three-leafed plants. The leaves are green and glossy. The edges can be smooth or jagged.

Poison sumac has many leaves growing off each stem.

All three plants have clusters of small, round, whitish-green flowers, which produce white berries. These appear in August or September and often remain through the winter.

When in doubt, stay away! Poison sumac has multiple leaves on each stem. It is even more difficult to detect since it can look like other, harmless types of sumac. All of these plants produce white berries. But the berries only grow during part of the year, so they're not a reliable warning sign.

The good news is that poison ivy doesn't grow everywhere in the continental United States. The bad news is that the places that don't have poison ivy (including parts of California) have poison oak. It's the same deal: same oil, same allergen, same reaction.

When it comes to poison ivy, oak, and sumac, the best advice is simple: Avoid them. That means wearing long pants, gloves, and long-sleeved shirts whenever you're in a place where they are. When you're finished outside, wash your clothes and hose off your tools to remove the oil. You might want to wash your dog, too: remember, his fur may hold the oil for days or weeks after he touches the plant.

Although wearing gloves is a far better choice, there are several "barrier" creams that can reduce your risk. Hydropel and Hollister Moisture Barrier are two products that you can rub on your hands and arms to help keep the oil away from your skin.

If you think you may have touched a plant, immediately wash off the area with soap and water. Better yet, apply rubbing alcohol to the suspected area. When even that fails and a rash develops, here are some tips for dealing with the itch.

- Try calamine lotion. This pink, milky solution can help dry out the blisters and sores. It may help with the itching, too.

- Over-the-counter hydrocortisone creams may also help. You apply these directly to the blistered areas.
- In more severe cases, see your doctor. You may need heavy-duty topical corticosteroids or even an oral prescription.
- No matter how much you want to, do not scratch the blisters. Scratching won't spread the rash, but it may cause an infection. Try covering the affected area with a gauze bandage at night so that you don't scratch in your sleep. If you do open up the rash by accident, wash it thoroughly and keep it covered with a loose, sterile bandage.

If you spot poison ivy growing in a place that you (or your pets) visit, it's best to remove the plants. Pulling them up won't always help because they can regrow from the roots. The best solution is to apply an herbicide, which kills the plant from the leaves down to the roots. When it dies, just let it be. Don't ever collect dead plants into a pile and burn them. If you breathe in the smoke, it can cause a severe rash inside your respiratory tract.

Other plants. Several other plants can cause reactions similar to poison ivy. They include ragweed (both the pollen and the plant itself can cause skin reactions), chrysanthemums, daisies, primrose, and wormwood. Southwesterners also may have to deal with sagebrush and heliotrope. In rare cases, some people may develop skin allergies to common foods like oranges, celery, and potatoes. As with poison ivy, avoidance is the best way to deal with these plants. If you don't touch them, they can't hurt you.

HIDDEN CAUSES

In many cases, it's easy to tell what is causing your skin to break out. For instance, some people with nickel allergies get a perfectly round rash on their wrist—right under the face of their watch. Not much doubt there.

But allergens can lurk everywhere, and they're not always easy to pinpoint. We've talked about the common allergens. Here are other substances that may cause skin reactions.

- *Medications.* These include antibiotic creams and ointments containing penicillin or sulfonamides, anesthetics (benzocaine), antihistamines, and antiseptics (hexachlorophene, thimerosal).
- *Formaldehyde.* This can appear in older types of home insulation and other building materials like particleboard. You'll also find formaldehyde in permanent press clothing. It's a good idea to wash new clothes several times before wearing them.
- *Cosmetics.* Everything from perfume to hair dye contains substances that can cause reactions. If you have skin allergies, it's always best to use hypoallergenic products.
- *Cleaning products.* Laundry soaps, dish detergents, and other common products often contain allergens.
- *Clothing.* Some clothes are treated with hydroquinone. This is usually applied to clothes with rubber or elastic parts, such as underwear and swimsuits.
- *Chemicals in the workplace.* These include chromates (which people who work with cement, electroplating, tanning, and paints can be exposed to), epoxy resins (plastics and construction workers), nickel salts (jewelers, cashiers), P-phenylenediamine (beauticians, mechanics), and many, many others.

If you can't easily spot the source of your skin allergies, try keeping a diary. Keep track of all the things that touch your skin, from soaps and clothes to plants and makeup. Make notes whenever you develop a rash. With a little luck, you may find your problem within a couple of weeks.

Then again, you might not. That's when it's time to see your doctor. After you describe the history of your problems, your doctor may be able to narrow the field of potential troublemakers. You may then take a patch test. This involves placing a small amount of an allergen on your skin to see if you have a reaction to it. While this isn't 100 percent reliable, it often can help identify the culprit. Then you'll have to talk with your doctor about the best ways to avoid touching the allergen—and how to deal with it when you make a mistake.

People with severe skin allergies should see their doctor immediately if they suspect a plant has touched sensitive areas like the eyelids and lips. These areas can swell drastically.

Nickel. In some people, this metal can cause a localized red, scaly rash that appears within hours after touching the skin. Unfortunately, nickel is everywhere these days—in zippers, buttons, watches, coins, pens, and especially jewelry. Even gold jewelry, unless it's 24-karat, may contain nickel to strengthen it.

If you get a rash in an area where metal touches skin—especially in pierced earlobes, under watches, or on your neckline—you probably are sensitive to nickel. It's best to avoid letting nickel touch your skin altogether.

That means you may want to switch to hypoallergenic stainless steel and silver jewelry. If you don't want to give up your favorite pieces, at least try dusting the skin with talcum powder before putting on the jewelry. This keeps the skin dry and may lessen your chances of developing a rash.

If you do develop a rash, the best treatment is a topical corticosteroid. You can get nonprescription-strength products at your local drugstore.

Latex rubber. Up until about 1980, this problem was hardly recognized. But since then, it's grown into a real concern. People use latex gloves for everything from surgery to food service. And balloons, rubber bands, shoe soles, condoms, and many other products contain latex, too. While only 1 percent of the population is sensitive to latex, the risk increases for health care workers; as many as 10 percent of them may be sensitized. And people who have other allergies seem to be at higher risk for being sensitive to latex.

Latex itself is only part of the problem. Gloves may be dusted with cornstarch or other materials to make them easier to take on and off. And other latex products, such as condoms, may be coated with gels that can cause the irritation.

Latex causes several reactions. The first is nonallergic. Even if you're not allergic to latex, it may cause dry, crusty lesions on your hands. In fact, this is the most common of all latex-related problems. Then there are the local allergic reactions, which are similar to the ones caused by poison ivy and nickel. In fact, the rashes that come from latex allergies look and feel very similar to poison ivy outbreaks.

The third type of reaction can be far more serious. In some cases, latex can cause whole-body allergic reactions. This can lead to relatively minor conditions like hives and swelling. But it also can trigger more severe reactions like asthma attacks or even anaphylaxis, a life-threatening response that can cause severe swelling of the throat, heart complications, and other serious problems. Anaphylaxis usually occurs only when a person is exposed to latex in sensitive areas, such as the chest cavity during surgery, the mouth during dental work, or the anus while receiving an enema. In some cases, however, just touching latex or breathing latex dust can trigger a reaction. If you know that you are extremely sensitive to latex and notice symptoms, see a doctor immediately.

Once again, avoidance is the best way to deal with latex allergies. But that may not always be possible. If you do touch latex and get a skin rash, topical corticosteroids may help relieve your symptoms. For whole-body reactions, including asthma, sneezing, or a runny nose, your doctor may recommend taking an antihistamine or a blast from a bronchodilator. If you know you're extremely sensitive, your doctor may give you a portable epinephrine kit for self-injections, which can stop anaphylactic reactions.

Photoallergic contact dermatitis. Most allergic skin reactions are straightforward: You touch the "wrong" thing—and pay the price. But sometimes just touching an allergen isn't enough to cause a rash. It's the combination of the allergen plus exposure to sunlight that leads to problems. This condition, called photoallergic contact dermatitis, is a particular problem with aftershave, perfume, sunscreens, and topical medications. In rare cases, eating certain foods (especially mangoes) can make your skin more sensitive to the allergen-sunlight combination.

Testing for this type of allergic reaction often includes a patch test. In addition, ultraviolet light will be applied briefly to the skin after the allergen patch is removed.

As always, the best way to avoid photoallergic problems is to avoid the allergen. If aftershave gives you a rash, don't use it. Or, if you can't stop using a product, you may be able to solve the problem by wearing sunblock with an SPF (sun protection factor) of 30 or higher. This will keep ultraviolet rays off your skin. If the sunblock itself causes the allergic reaction, try switching to a non-PABA sunblock. Often, PABA is the key allergen in sunblock products.

Contact urticaria. Most skin allergies cause an itchy, ugly rash. But if you have a condition called contact urticaria, you may get hives or welts instead. These are pink or red raised patches on the skin, ranging in size from half an inch to nearly 12 inches. The rash can last as little as an hour or as long as a day. Hives are very common. About one in five people will get hives sometime in their lives.

Hives can be caused by allergies to food, especially shellfish, milk, nuts, and eggs, and by pet dander, dust, and pollen. But hives also may be caused by direct skin contact with allergens. Either way, the reaction is the same. Hives are believed to be caused by the release of histamine. That makes them different from most skin allergies, which are caused by T-cell reactions.

Here's a list of potential allergens that can cause hives when they touch skin: sunscreen ingredients, hair spray, nickel, perfume, birch wood, milk, menthol, nail polish, and medicines like bacitracin, neomycin, and benzoyl peroxide. Workers who handle animal proteins, food proteins (in flour, grain, and spices), and latex proteins (those who use or make latex gloves) are at higher risk of developing allergic contact urticarias.

Once again, patch tests can sometimes help identify the cause of a hives outbreak. But before it comes to that, you may be able to discover the cause by keeping a diary of things that touched your skin prior to an outbreak. Once you have an outbreak, you can treat hives with topical corticosteroid creams or oral antihistamines. In severe cases, your doctor may prescribe an oral corticosteroid such as prednisone.

HOW IRRITATING!

Earlier in this chapter we mentioned that most skin rashes are not caused by allergies. Instead, they're triggered by **irritants**—substances that cause redness, swelling, burns, blisters, and other problems when they touch the skin. Because they're such a wide-ranging group, these irritants work in many different ways. But the thing they have in common is that there's no T-cell allergic reaction behind the rash.

You don't have to go through a sensitization process to develop "irritant contact dermatitis." The first time you touch an irritant you can have problems. With some substances, however, it may take years of low-level exposure before the trouble starts.

Here's a list of common skin irritants.

- Paints and solvents, including alcohol and turpentine
- Acids
- Cement
- Lime (calcium oxide)
- Some plastics and metals
- Alkalis, like lye and drain cleaner

Even soaps can cause problems. That's because they remove the natural oils from your skin, leaving it dry, brittle, and easily irritated by other substances. While this is not an excuse for your kids to stop washing their hands, it is a good reason for you to keep plenty of hand creams and moisturizing soaps around the house.

In general, places on your body with thin skin are more vulnerable to irritation. That includes your face and eyelids, and the genital area.

In many cases, finding out what's causing the irritation is easy. If you dip your hands in paint thinner and don't use gloves, it's pretty simple to figure out what caused the rash. But we touch so many things every day that sometimes it's hard to spot a single cause. As with allergic skin conditions, keeping a diary can help. If the problem persists, your doctor may be able to help with patch tests. As always, the only way to keep the rash from returning is to avoid touching the irritants.

ECZEMA: THE MYSTERY RASH

We're going to end our discussion of skin problems by talking about a condition that's part allergy and part mystery. It's called atopic dermatitis, or eczema. People with eczema often have red, scaly, brittle, itchy patches of skin. Most of these patches are on the scalp, face, arms, and legs—especially on joints like elbows and knees. While 1 in 10 children and infants has eczema, most eventually outgrow the problem. Still, about 3 percent of adults have a lingering case.

Just what causes eczema remains a mystery. Doctors know that it's somehow related to allergies. In fact, 70 percent of people with eczema conditions have a family history of either asthma, allergic rhinitis (hay fever), or eczema. Most have high levels of immunoglobulin E (IgE) in their bloodstream. And one-third of people with eczema will eventually develop hay fever or asthma themselves.

Unfortunately, there's no cure for eczema yet. But there are lots of ways to cut down on the outbreaks.

Play it cool. Taking short, cool showers will help prevent dry skin. Children should not get more than three baths per week, because too much water can dry the skin.

Use a mild soap when you bathe, such as Dove or Eucerin. Use the soap only on your groin area and under your arms. You can clean the rest of your body with a nonperfumed bath oil. When you're taking a bath instead of a shower, add the non-perfumed bath oil to water. Then gently sponge your body. AlphaKeri and Domol are good products for this.

When you've finished showering, gently pat yourself dry. Don't rub with the towel.

Take care of your skin. Use plenty of moisturizer. Face creams, hand creams, petroleum jelly, and even regular cooking oil will help lube up those dry spots. Eucerin, Pond's, Vaseline, and Nivea are common brands of moisturizers that may help.

Put water, water everywhere. In most cases, too much humidity in the house can cause problems. It can lead to mold growth, which is a big problem for people with allergies. But people with eczema should consider using a humidifier, at least in their bedroom. You can also put a pan of water near the radiator to moisten the air. This will help keep the skin moist and protected.

Avoid your triggers. For many people, especially children, eating certain foods can make eczema worse. Many of these are the same bad guys that cause food allergies. They include egg whites, dairy products, fish and shellfish, wheat products, and oranges. If you think that food may be causing a problem for you, try a little experimenting. Keep a food diary, listing what you ate over a two- or three-week period and noting how your eczema reacted. You may spot the troublemaker by yourself. If not, consult your doctor. He might decide to put you on an elimination diet, which cuts out foods one at a time until the problem is resolved. We'll talk more about food and allergies in the next chapter.

If you have large patches of eczema that start to weep, you can try taking a lukewarm bath using Aveeno moisturizer with colloidal oatmeal. About one-half cup will do. For smaller areas, try mixing a teaspoon of table salt into one pint of cool water. Dab the water onto the affected skin with cotton balls.

Try to avoid scratching patches of dry skin. If things get so bad that you have trouble resisting, run cold water over the affected area. You can also use an ice bag to dull the itch.

CHAPTER 5

Food Allergies: Find Out What's Eating You

We all know what it's like to have a good meal go bad. The waitress hasn't even cleared the dessert dishes when the feeling starts. An uneasy rumble in the belly, followed by a little queasiness. By the time you pay the check, you're feeling nauseated. And just as you pull into the driveway your body decides it needs to get rid of that fancy food fast—one way or another.

It's one of the worst feelings in the world. But is it really an allergy? In most cases, probably not. Ninety-nine times out of a hundred, bad reactions to food are caused by other reasons, such as food poisoning or a simple food intolerance. Many of the symptoms are the same: diarrhea, upset stomach, abdominal pain, vomiting. Yet knowing the subtle differences between allergies and other food-related problems can be very important. In extreme cases, it may even save your life.

Let's take a few minutes to talk about true food allergies and how to find out what's really causing that bellyache.

A BELLYFUL OF TROUBLE

Allergic reactions are always caused by allergens—tiny, usually harmless substances that your immune system mistakes for dangerous invaders. Your body overreacts to these allergens and gives them the same nasty treatment that it usually reserves for viruses and germs. That's what causes all the symptoms.

When you breathe, allergens like mold spores, dust mite excretions, and pollen can enter your nose and lungs. When you eat, allergens (usually proteins in food) go down the hatch and into your digestive system. Either way, the reaction is pretty much the same. The allergens in your stomach are absorbed into the bloodstream, where they meet the immune system. When you encounter a food allergen for the first time, your immune system reacts by producing large amounts of immunoglobulin E (IgE) antibodies. These antibodies are specific to the allergen; for example, the antibodies for peanut proteins will not react to parsley proteins.

You're now sensitized to the food allergen. This means that the next time you eat that food, your body is armed for a fight. The antibodies have attached themselves to giant mast cells, which are full of histamine and other chemicals. When the antibody spots its particular allergen, it grabs onto it—and triggers the mast cell to release its contents.

The symptoms you feel depend on where your antibodies run into the allergens. Digestion is a very complicated process, involving many parts of your body. The first place you come into contact with the food (unless you spill some on yourself first) is your mouth. When you chew, the allergen may be detected by antibodies and mast cells in the tissues of your tongue or cheeks. So, shortly after you take your first mouthful, you may feel a tingling sensation.

When you swallow, food passes down the esophagus. There it can trigger reactions that can cause more tingling—in your throat—and perhaps even a feeling of tightness. The third stop is the stomach and intestines. Here the allergic reaction can result in abdominal pain, diarrhea, or vomiting. When the allergens get absorbed through the intestines and into the bloodstream, they can travel all over your body. When they reach your lungs, they can cause difficulty breathing—even asthma in people who are prone to attacks. Eventually, the allergens may make it to your skin, where the allergic reaction can cause hives or eczema.

It doesn't take long for all this to happen—as little as a few minutes to an hour. The good news is that, with rare but important exceptions, the discomfort will pass as soon as your body has rid itself of the allergen. That's usually a matter of hours.

Many foods can cause allergic reactions. But more than 90 percent of reactions are caused by eight types of food.

- Shellfish, including crab, lobster, and crayfish
- Fish
- Egg and egg products
- Nuts from trees, including walnuts
- Peanuts
- Wheat and wheat products
- Milk and milk products
- Soy and soy products

FOOD INTOLERANCE

About 40 percent of American adults believe they have a food allergy. In truth, that number is much lower—probably about 1 percent. So what's causing all the digestive distress in the world? Well, lots of things. Unlike food allergies, food intolerances don't involve the immune system. But they can make you just as miserable as true allergies, causing such things as diarrhea, vomiting, and skin rashes. In fact, without talking to a doctor or taking some tests, it may be almost impossible for you to tell the difference between an allergy and an intolerance.

Here's a look at some of the most common food intolerances.

Lactase deficiency. Some people don't have the stomach for milk. This is because milk contains a substance called lactose, which as many as 10 percent of adults can't digest. To digest lactose, you need an enzyme called lactase. If you don't produce enough lactase, the lactose in dairy foods just stays around in your digestive tract. Eventually, it may get used by bacteria that line your intestines. This can cause some uncomfortable problems like gas, bloating, or diarrhea. People from certain racial groups are more likely than others to have lactase deficiency. These include Asians (as many as 90 percent have some degree of deficiency) and both blacks and American Indians (75 percent).

Food additives. Years ago, a loaf of bread was nothing more than flour, yeast, and maybe a few nuts to make things crunchy. Today, you need a doctorate in chemistry to read the package; bread is often full of stabilizers, colors, artificial flavors, preservatives, and other space-age stuff. Well, these additives can give some people fits. Here are the major troublemakers.

- *Monosodium glutamate (MSG).* This is a flavor enhancer that's frequently used in Asian cooking. In large amounts, it can cause a wide range of problems, from headaches and nausea to tightness in the chest.
- *Nitrates and nitrites.* These are preservatives that are often found in processed meats like salami and hot dogs. They can cause headaches and possibly hives.
- *Sulfites.* These are also preservatives, frequently found in beers and wines, cookies and crackers, and canned and bottled foods. They formerly were used to keep vegetables crisp in salad bars, but the Food and Drug Administration put a stop to that when too many people had bad reactions. Symptoms include hives, cramps, diarrhea, and headaches. Some people with asthma may suffer attacks when they eat sulfites.
- *BHA and BHT.* These are used to keep cereals and other grain products fresh-tasting. They can rarely cause skin reactions.
- *Aspartame.* This is a low-calorie sweetener better known by its brand name, NutraSweet. In rare cases it can cause hives or swelling of the hands and feet.
- *Parabens.* These are preservatives, including the common ingredient sodium benzoate. In some people, parabens can cause skin rashes.
- *Food dyes.* These are commonly suspected but rarely proved to be the cause of food reactions.

Natural substances. Many foods don't need additives to cause problems. Some contain histamines, the same chemicals that mast cells release during an allergic reaction. If you eat foods with a high histamine content, you could develop symptoms that mimic those of allergies: stomach cramps, vomiting, and so on.

Fermented foods often have lots of histamines. These include wine, fermented cheeses (like Swiss cheese), and sauerkraut. Dried meats and canned fish like anchovies also contain histamines. Tuna and mackerel are two of the main histamine-filled foods.

It's not just histamine that causes problems, however. Food ingredients ranging from caffeine to cocoa can create digestive trouble. The list is a long one, but the main offenders include chocolate, cola, coffee, tea, beer, vinegar, yeast, bananas, citrus fruits, and avocados.

Children are especially likely to have allergies to fish, eggs, and milk. Both children and adults are more likely to be allergic to foods that they eat most often. In Japan, for example, allergic reactions to rice are more common than in places where less rice is consumed. The same is true of deepwater fish like cod in Scandinavian countries.

Here's another interesting allergy tidbit: Researchers don't know why, but when you were born may determine whether you developed food allergies as a child. A Swedish study of more than 200 children found that those born between September and February were much more likely than others to develop IgE antibodies to egg whites, milk, and wheat products. They also were more likely to develop eczema.

FOOD POISONING

Food poisoning is different from food intolerance. Intolerances are caused by substances that naturally occur in foods or are intentionally added to them. Food poisoning is caused by organisms that have infected a food, like *Salmonella* bacteria. Food can be tainted by improper handling, poor refrigeration, insects, and other things. Polluted water can affect foods. Even something as bizarre as a steer eating poisonous plants before being butchered can cause trouble.

Unlike food allergies or intolerances, food poisoning usually takes a while to develop. Instead of feeling symptoms in minutes, you may not feel the worst of food poisoning for hours, or even a day or two. And unless you continue getting your food from the same contaminated source, food poisoning is usually a one-shot deal. Eating tainted potato salad once won't make you allergic to, or intolerant of, potato salad forever.

OTHER PROBLEMS

Sometimes people develop temporary sensitivity to foods. A child who has a viral infection, for example, may become intolerant of milk for a while. If you have ulcers, cancer, or other internal problems, you may become sensitive to foods that didn't bother you before. The same goes for people who are taking medications, including drugs used to treat depression, like monoamine oxidase inhibitors.

In a few cases, psychological problems can cause bad reactions to food. People who associate a particular food with a bad episode in their lives may develop symptoms that mimic those of an allergic reaction when they eat the food. This often requires some form of therapy to overcome.

DOING A LITTLE DETECTIVE WORK

Remember the old joke about the guy who went to see the doctor because he had a pain in his neck? "It hurts when I do this," he says, turning his head sharply to one side.

"Then stop doing it," the doctor tells him.

You cure food allergies the same way: If you get sick whenever you eat a certain food, don't eat it. This is the only way to deal with a food allergy or intolerance. There's no magic pill, no secret treatment. If peanuts make you sick, you'll just have to snack on pretzels instead.

Of course, this assumes that you know which food is causing the trouble. It's not always so easy. If you break out in hives every time you eat lobster, that's pretty clear-cut. But what if you're allergic to something less obvious? Or what if you have reactions only after you've eaten a certain amount of an allergen? Or what if you have reactions only on certain occasions when you eat a food? In tougher cases, it's going to require some time and a little discipline on your part. It may also require a trip to a specialist to finally track down the source of your trouble.

You can begin on your own by keeping a food diary. This really isn't hard. Just write down the foods you eat at each meal. Make sure that you note the time you eat. After eating, keep a close watch on your reactions. If you develop any of the telltale symptoms of allergy or intolerance within an hour or two, make a note.

When you do have a reaction, write down the contents of the foods you ate. If it's something you cooked, note the ingredients you used. If it is a packaged food, save the label. Sooner or later you may notice a pattern. Maybe you get reactions after eating foods made with egg whites. Or maybe it is a food additive that keeps showing up on your list. Once you think you've spotted a suspect, try to avoid eating the food or additive for a while. If you don't have any more symptoms, you may have solved the mystery by yourself.

You may not be so lucky, however. If you keep having symptoms and can't pinpoint the source within a couple of weeks, it's time to see a doctor. Allergy specialists are trained to spot hard-to-identify food allergies and intolerances, and their experience can save you countless hours of digestive agony.

The first thing a doctor will do is ask about your history of food reactions. She will want to know how long you've been having problems. Do the symptoms arrive quickly, or are they delayed more than an hour after eating? Do you cook your food thoroughly, or do you like rare or raw foods? (Sometimes cooking can destroy allergens.) Did other people who ate the same foods also get sick? Do you exercise immediately after eating? (Some people develop reactions only if they exercise following a meal.) Are the reactions worse at a certain time of the year? (Some people who are allergic to ragweed pollen have allergic reactions to melons only when pollen counts are high.) You'll answer a whole bunch of questions that may uncover the cause of your reactions right away.

If not, it may be time to go back to the diet diary. Perhaps your doctor's trained eye will be able to spot the culprit when you couldn't. Once your doctor believes she's found a possible suspect, she may start you on what's called an **elimination diet**. You'll avoid eating foods that contain the possible troublemaker to see if your reactions go away. If they do, then your doctor will tell you to try eating the suspect food again to see if the reactions return. If they do, it's probably a pretty good bet that you've identified your problem. Reintroducing the food should be done only under a doctor's supervision, especially if you've had strong reactions in the past.

If your doctor is confident that your problem is solved, that may be the end of the tests. But if there's still a little room for doubt, there are other procedures to try. The first is **skin tests**. A diluted amount of the suspected allergen is placed on your skin, usually somewhere on your arm. The skin is then scratched or punctured gently so that the allergen can react with your body. If you develop redness or swelling in the area, you probably have IgE antibodies in your system for that allergen.

Skin tests are fast and simple. But they're not 100 percent reliable. Just because you have a skin reaction doesn't mean you'll have a reaction when you eat the allergen. It's a judgment call that your doctor makes based on your history and previous tests.

Alternatively, you'll have a blood test to check for the presence of particular antibodies in your bloodstream. The two most common tests, and the most reliable, are the **RAST** (radioallergosorbent test) and **ELISA** (enzyme-linked immunosorbent assay). Both tests can consistently spot IgE antibodies. But, as with skin tests, just having the antibody doesn't mean you necessarily have a food allergy. Blood tests also tend to be more expensive than skin tests, and results can take a couple of days to a week to get back to your doctor.

The final method of testing is called a **double-blind food challenge**. This is considered by many experts to be the most reliable test of all. During the test, a person takes capsules that contain different food extracts. Some of the extracts are suspected of being allergens for the person, while others are not. The doctor notes whether the patient has any reactions to each capsule. Neither the doctor nor the patient knows which capsules are which until after the test—that's why it's called double-blind.

The food challenge is an excellent way to pinpoint specific food allergies. It can also rule out certain foods that a person may feel are causing his trouble. But this test is not for everybody. If you have severe reactions to food allergens, taking capsules full of them is not a good idea. And the test can be expensive and time-consuming.

If you feel that you need an allergy doctor to help you with your food problems, read chapter 8, where we'll talk about finding a physician who's right for you.

As with all allergies, the best way to deal with food allergies or intolerances is to avoid the food that's causing your problems. If you're cooking at home, that's pretty easy. About the only tricky part is reading labels on packaged foods. If you know that you have bad reactions to a food additive, check the packaging to make sure that it's not in the products you use. The federal government requires food manufacturers to list all ingredients. But the list can be pretty long sometimes, so read carefully.

Allergens can hide in the darnedest foods. Here are some surprising places you might find them.

Milk: Deli meats, soft-serve ice cream (even non-dairy types), creamed soups and sauces, tuna fish salad, margarine. If you see a "D" on the product label, that means it has milk proteins in it.

Eggs: Baked goods, mayonnaise, noodles. Even egg substitutes can contain egg whites.

Wheat: Noodles, gravies, ice cream. Labels that say "natural flavors" may indicate the presence of wheat products.

Peanuts: Pie crusts, Mexican dishes, Thai dishes. Peanut butter is even used to thicken chili and to seal the end of Chinese egg rolls.

Other nuts: Salad dressings, muffins, barbecue and other savory sauces.

Because of increased demand from consumers, more manufacturers are producing food substitutes. These can be used in place of common foods—like milk, eggs, and wheat—that often cause problems. To find out more about these products, check the appendix in the back of this book.

Whenever you eat out, you're rolling the dice a little with food allergies. You must ask whether the dish you want contains the food that you're allergic to. Don't take "I don't know" for an answer. Politely explain that you have an allergy to certain foods.

If you get a bad reaction from monosodium glutamate (MSG), by all means ask the chef to prepare your meal without it. That's especially important with Chinese food, which often contains MSG. In fact, intolerance to MSG is sometimes called Chinese Restaurant Syndrome.

Once in a while, an allergen may slip past you and cause a mild reaction. When that happens, treat the itching and swelling with an over-the-counter antihistamine. This will help blunt your body's response and make you feel better faster. There's a list of antihistamine medicines on page 156. If you have an asthma attack, use your bronchodilator to help ease your reaction. Intestinal symptoms will get better over time.

Unfortunately, you can't prevent food allergies by taking medication ahead of time. Medication only works once an allergic reaction is under way.

ANAPHYLAXIS: A DEADLY THREAT

It's hard to tell the difference between a true food allergy and food intolerance. And in many cases, it really doesn't matter much. Both of them can make you feel lousy, and the best way to deal with both is to avoid eating the foods that cause trouble.

But there's one case in which the difference can literally mean life or death. In very rare cases, food allergies can spin out of control and lead to a condition called anaphylaxis.

Anaphylaxis starts like other allergic reactions: IgE antibodies find an allergen in the body and the immune system starts its misguided work. But it doesn't stop with sneezing or hives or an upset stomach. When the allergen causes your body to release massive amounts of histamines and other chemicals, your blood vessels can open wide and cause a sharp drop in blood pressure.

As you can see, this is serious business. The reaction can affect many parts of your body, including your lungs

SYMPTOMS OF ANAPHYLACTIC SHOCK

Anaphylaxis is the most serious of all allergic reactions. Unless treated immediately, it can lead to serious complications—even death. Any number of allergens can trigger an anaphylactic reaction, including foods, bee stings, and drugs. Here are the typical symptoms of anaphylaxis:

- Swelling in the lips, tongue, throat, hands, or feet, usually accompanied by itching.
- Tingling sensations in the mouth and on the face
- Difficulty breathing, shortness of breath, coughing, wheezing, and/or hoarseness
- Nasal congestion, usually with sneezing and itching
- Chest pain or tightness
- Change in voice or difficulty swallowing
- Warm sensation or flushing, redness of the skin, sometimes with hives, swelling, and severe itching. (In the case of bee stings, these can occur in areas far from the site of the actual sting.)
- Dizziness and lightheadedness, and even possible loss of consciousness, due to a drop in blood pressure.
- Nausea, vomiting, diarrhea, or abdominal cramps
- Feelings of anxiety or sense of impending doom

If you notice any of these symptoms, contact a doctor or go to the emergency room immediately. You will most likely need an injection of epinephrine to relieve the symptoms.

and heart. Without prompt treatment, anaphylaxis can damage major organs in your body. It can even be fatal.

Fortunately, the odds of having an anaphylactic reaction are low. The average person has about a 1 percent chance over a lifetime. The bad part is that no one can tell who's going to have one. You're at higher risk if you have severe allergies, but it can happen to anyone. One recent study found that women may be twice as likely to suffer an anaphylactic reaction as men. No one knows why this may be so.

Many allergens can trigger anaphylaxis, including bee or wasp stings and drugs like penicillin, seizure medications, and muscle relaxants. Food allergies, however, may be the most common cause. The trigger foods for anaphylaxis are the same ones that cause regular food allergies: peanuts, milk, shellfish, fish, and eggs. Certain vegetables, like celery, also can spur a reaction.

In highly sensitive people, tiny amounts of food allergens can result in anaphylaxis. Researchers have found that .002 percent of a peanut kernel may trigger a reaction. You can barely see that small an amount, let alone taste it.

The point here is not to get you scared. It's to alert you to the problem. If you feel the symptoms of anaphylaxis after eating, get to a doctor or emergency room immediately.

Treatment for anaphylaxis usually involves getting an injection of epinephrine, also known as adrenaline. If you have a history of anaphylaxis, your doctor probably will give you a portable epinephrine kit. The most common brand is called an EpiPen. It's a tiny needle that you use to inject yourself if you feel an anaphylactic

ALLERGY SAFETY AT SCHOOL

Approximately 50 insect-sting deaths and 100 food-allergy deaths occur in the United States each year. If your child has allergies, he or she could face a life-threatening situation. Although you know what to do in an emergency, what happens when you're not around? What about when your child's at school?

The American Academy of Allergy, Asthma and Immunology (AAAAI) recommends that all schools be prepared to act if a student suffers a severe allergic reaction while at school. Following are some ways your child's school can prepare itself for such an event:

- Have a physician prescribe an appropriate treatment protocol for the school's use.
- Before each school year begins, parents of a child with allergies should discuss the situation with school officials. It's critical that the school be made aware of the potentially life-threatening consequences of an unexpected allergic reaction, if your child is at risk of food or insect sting anaphylaxis.
- Include in the child's file an identification sheet with his or her name, photograph, specific allergy (e.g., peanut or bee sting), warning signs of reactions, and the proper emergency treatment. Make sure this information is readily retrievable by all school staff. It should not, for confidentiality reasons, be available to other parents or students.
- While school staff should ensure that the child avoids potential allergy-causing situations, they should help the child lead as normal a school life as possible.

- Make sure that all school staff members know which children have allergies that may need to be treated by epinephrine (adrenaline). If a doctor prescribes an epinephrine auto-injector device for a particular student, the staff should be aware of this and should know where to retrieve the device in case of emergency. Each auto-injector should be clearly labeled with the child's name and classroom number. Expiration dates on the devices should be checked regularly.
- Whenever possible, children with food allergies—especially children in nursery schools—should wear some form of identification, e.g., a Medic Alert bracelet, necklace, or badge. For ordering information, call (800) 432-5398, or write to: Medic Alert, 2323 Colorado Ave., Turlock, CA, 95380.
- School staff who serve food or who supervise eating times should know the ingredients of the foods they serve to children with allergies.
- A rule stating that no food or utensils can be traded with any other student should be strictly enforced for food-allergic children.
- All surfaces—tables, toys, countertops, dishes—should be washed well, expecially when used by children under three. If these are mouthed by toddlers, even tiny traces of a food allergen can cause an allergic reaction.
- Avoid using foods to which a student is allergic as part of a lesson plan, e.g., for science, crafts, or cooking classes.
- Encourage regular hand-washing after eating for everyone.

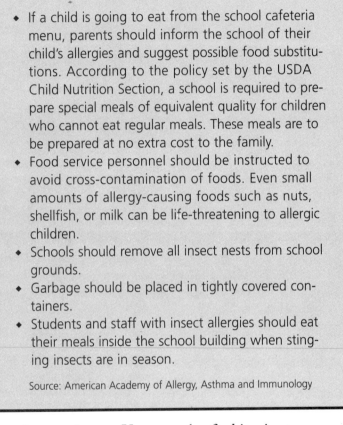

- If a child is going to eat from the school cafeteria menu, parents should inform the school of their child's allergies and suggest possible food substitutions. According to the policy set by the USDA Child Nutrition Section, a school is required to prepare special meals of equivalent quality for children who cannot eat regular meals. These meals are to be prepared at no extra cost to the family.
- Food service personnel should be instructed to avoid cross-contamination of foods. Even small amounts of allergy-causing foods such as nuts, shellfish, or milk can be life-threatening to allergic children.
- Schools should remove all insect nests from school grounds.
- Garbage should be placed in tightly covered containers.
- Students and staff with insect allergies should eat their meals inside the school building when stinging insects are in season.

Source: American Academy of Allergy, Asthma and Immunology

reaction coming on. You may also find it wise to wear a Medic Alert bracelet warning doctors about your condition. This is especially true if you have severe allergies to drugs like penicillin. We'll talk about this more in chapter 7.

KIDS AND FOOD ALLERGIES

While food allergies are literally a one-in-a-hundred occurrence in adults, kids aren't quite so lucky. As many as 3 percent of children may have true allergic reactions to food. This may be because kids' immune and digestive systems are not yet up to full speed. Many children outgrow allergies, especially to milk and soy products. Allergies to shellfish, fish, or peanuts, however, are more likely to stay with a child for life.

The symptoms of allergic reactions to food are usually the same in children as they are in adults. But infants may develop colic instead or have blood in their stools. Newborns can have allergic reactions to cow's milk and soy early in life. Because it's tough to tell exactly what's causing the problem, it's very important that you report these reactions to your pediatrician immediately.

If cow's milk turns out to be the cause, you have a few options. Mothers can try breast-feeding or using a soy-based formula. If soy also causes trouble, your doctor may recommend elemental formulas. These are made of sugars and amino acids that rarely cause allergic reactions.

There's no hard evidence that breast-feeding your baby will prevent future allergies to food. But if breast milk is all that your child eats, then at least allergies to milk, soy, and other foods won't develop during the infant's first months of life. There's only one exception: Some children have such strong food allergies that they have a reaction to breast milk if the mother has been eating the problem food. If that's the case, your doctor will tell you to avoid that food until breast-feeding ends.

There's no proof that avoiding certain foods during pregnancy can prevent allergies in babies. So don't skimp on milk and other foods while you're carrying your child. You and your baby need full, balanced nutrition, and these foods are unlikely to cause problems in any event.

CHAPTER 6

Insect Bites and Stings: Bee Alert!

Sometimes we can't leave things well enough alone. Take those bees in the backyard. They were just doing bee things: making honey, carrying pollen, and buzzing around your open can of orange soda just in case it needed pollinating.

But you swatted down their nest anyway—and then you ended up with a few stinging reminders about why you shouldn't mess around with Mother Nature.

If you're like most people, occasional insect stings are nothing more than a nuisance, although sometimes a painful one. They swell up, hurt and itch for a while, and then disappear. But for an estimated two million Americans, they can be a lot more dangerous. Allergic reactions to bees, wasps, hornets, and fire ants can cause severe reactions, including deadly anaphylaxis. An average of about 50 people a year die in this country as a result of insect stings.

In this chapter we'll talk about how to avoid stings in the first place. Then we'll look at the warning signs of an allergic reaction and tell you what to do when you think things are getting out of control.

DANGEROUS REACTIONS

In North America, there are two kinds of bugs to worry about. One type bites you so that it can feed on your blood. These bugs include ticks, chiggers, fleas, mosquitoes, and lice. They're sneaky little creatures. They get on your skin when you're not paying attention. When they bite, they inject an anticoagulant that makes it easier for them to have a meal. Then they fall off or fly away, usually leaving you with a raised, itchy lump.

These bites are unpleasant and irritating but are unlikely to cause allergic reactions. Much more dangerous are stinging insects like wasps, hornets, honeybees, yellow jackets, and fire ants. These bugs aren't sneaky at all. They don't want anything from you except a little room to operate. In fact, the only reason they're interested in you at all is because you pose a threat to them. You might not see it that way, but look at it from the insect's point of view. There's Mr. Honeybee, minding his own business, collecting pollen from a field of clover, and here you come with your lawnmower, a can of bug spray, or a giant, nest-bashing stick.

These insects sting you as a warning to stay away. They defend their territory by poking you with a sharp little needle. If you're smart, you get the point immediately and get away from the nest. If not, you're likely to get stung numerous times until the lesson sinks in.

The insects inject venom into your skin. In most people, this poison causes a couple of reactions. First, it makes the area around the sting hurt. Next, it can cause the area to swell up and turn red. The venom also may cause itching. These are **local reactions** that don't appear anywhere except the area immediately surrounding the sting.

If you're allergic, however, the effects can travel through your entire body. You might develop hives on your back, even though the wasp stung your foot. You may notice redness and swelling in other parts of your body, too. And in severe cases, you can develop the telltale signs of anaphylaxis: swelling in the throat, difficulty breathing, low blood pressure, nausea, and other symptoms. (See the box on page 90.) These are called **systemic reactions** because they occur all over your body.

The mechanisms involved in allergic reactions to insect stings are pretty much the same as those in hay fever. When your immune system discovers an allergen, specific antibodies (made of immunoglobulin E, or IgE) grab it and bind it to mast cells or basophils. These cells then release their toxic chemicals, including histamine, to kill the intruder. The result is an allergic reaction that ranges from hives to asthma. It's important to note that it's not the toxins in the bee venom that cause the problem. It's particular proteins included in the venom. The venom itself was designed to leave you only with a little welt, not a body-wide allergic reaction.

As with many other allergic reactions, you have to be sensitized to the allergen before it causes problems. You won't get hay fever the first time you breathe ragweed pollen, and you won't have an allergic reaction to a bee sting the first time you get zapped. That's because your immune system must first build up its IgE antibodies against the allergen. After those antibodies are present, any exposure to the allergen can result in a reaction.

What separates bee stings from hay fever is the severity of the reaction and the route the allergen takes into the body. While only one person in a hundred is at risk for insect-sting allergies, the potential problems the reaction can cause are severe—even life-threatening. Within minutes of being stung, your body can begin to develop the signs of an anaphylactic reaction. If you or someone you are with has been stung, it is imperative that you are alert to the signs of anaphylactic shock. These are detailed in the box, "Symptoms of Anaphylactic Shock" on page 90.

If you notice any of these symptoms after getting stung, seek medical help immediately. Anaphylaxis is not something to mess around with. In severe cases, it can lead to cardiac arrest and even death. And there's no way for you to predict how you're going to react. So always err on the side of safety and seek emergency help right away.

PROTECTIVE MEASURES

Insects sting you to defend themselves. They're usually not going to bother you if you don't egg them on. So the best way to avoid insect sting allergies is to avoid the insects. It's not that hard to do. Here's how.

Don't dress like a flower. Bees are attracted to bright, vibrant colors. It's nature's way of saying, "Pollen for sale." If you decide to do the yard work wearing a Hawaiian flower shirt, yellow shorts, and orange sneakers, you're asking for trouble. It's best to dress in more muted hues: tans, browns, or black—the colors of dirt. Bees aren't very interested in dirt.

Don't smell like a flower either. Your husband loves the smell of your perfume, so why wouldn't a wasp? Insects instinctively follow sweet aromas, since they usually mean there's pollen nearby. When you go on a picnic or do some yard work, skip the Eau de Honeysuckle. You'll only be wasting it on a bunch of hornets.

Unfortunately, smelling bad won't keep stinging insects away, either. Bug repellent works only on biting insects, which want to eat your blood. Bees, hornets, and fire ants sting because you're messing with their turf. They don't care how awful you smell.

Wear shoes. Walking barefoot through the clover is one of the rites of summer. Sadly, it's also one of the best ways to get stung. Clover flowers are a honeybee favorite. Since the flowers are so low to the ground, you're not likely to notice a bee until you step on it. If you're wearing sneakers, well, it's bye-bye bee. But if you're barefoot, that bee may decide to plant its stinger in your sole.

Keep a lid on it: Part I. Bees like food smells as much as they like perfume. If you're eating on the deck or having a picnic, be sure to keep your food covered as much as possible. This includes drinks like lemonade and sugary sodas; bees often crawl inside the cans for a drink. You know how much a sting on the neck hurts— imagine one inside your mouth!

Keep a lid on it: Part II. Bees are as attracted to your table scraps as they are to the main course. So when you're finished with that picnic, seal the garbage in a plastic bag and drop it in a covered trash can.

Don't wait, exterminate. Bees, hornets, and wasps are useful creatures. They pollinate plants and help rid

ZAPPED!

No matter how careful we are, a bee's going to get our number once in a while. We might be raking leaves, walking down a country lane, or just sitting on a sun porch when it happens. If you do get stung, remain calm. And watch for symptoms. The least you're going to notice is a red, swollen area around the sting. That's a local reaction, and it's perfectly normal. What you're on the alert for is a systemic, or whole-body, reaction. If you notice hives forming on a spot far away from the sting, you're having an allergic reaction. If you notice any of the other signs of anaphylaxis (see "Symptoms of Anaphylactic Shock" on page 90), things may be about to get pretty hairy.

Any time you notice the slightest sign of an allergic reaction to a bee sting, get to a doctor. Severe reactions may start with just an itchy throat or a rash, but within minutes you could develop full-blown anaphylaxis. We can't stress this enough: Don't take allergic reactions to bee stings lightly. Seek emergency help immediately.

Once you've shown signs of bee-sting allergies, your doctor will probably give you a kit that includes an emergency injection tube called an EpiPen. This contains epinephrine, a form of adrenaline that works quickly to stop allergic reactions. It constricts blood vessels, relaxes the muscles in the lungs, reduces swelling, and stimulates your heartbeat. It's important that you carry this medicine with you at all times. Because once you've had an episode—even a mild one—you're much more likely to have a similar or even worse reaction the next time you get stung.

The EpiPen is easy to use. You just push it against your thigh and press a button. It's pretty much painless, so don't worry about that. You should notice relief from your symptoms almost immediately.

Keep in mind that the EpiPen is emergency medicine. Once you've used it, you still need to get to the doctor right away. For one thing, the effects of the epinephrine may wear off within 20 minutes or so. And one dose may not be enough to fight off all the dangerous symptoms—especially if you get stung more than once.

Try to identify the insect that stung you and tell your doctor. Was it a honeybee, yellow jacket, hornet, wasp, or fire ant? They all have slightly different venoms, and you may not be allergic to all of them. Also, a honeybee leaves its barbed stinger in your skin before it flies off and dies. This stinger is a hollow, barbed needle that probably still contains some venom. It's important to remove the stinger without releasing any more venom into your body. To do this, take a dull table knife or a credit card and place it against your skin and the stinger. Scrape across your skin to remove the stinger. Don't use tweezers because they may squeeze more venom into your skin.

your garden of unwanted pests. But when they decide to build their dream nest too close to yours, it's time to take action. If you are allergic to insect venom, call an exterminator to get rid of nests and colonies. Don't take any chances with getting stung.

If the nest is located in a remote corner of your yard, it may not be worth the effort. Just don't venture near it. Stinging insects are at their angriest when they think you're messing with their nest. This is especially important during summer and early fall, when bees are their busiest. At these times, large nests can contain more than 60,000 insects.

DON'T BE SO SENSITIVE

There's no true cure for bee-sting allergies. But there is one method that may greatly reduce your chances of having a reaction the next time you get zapped. It's called immunotherapy. Over the course of weeks, months, or perhaps years, an allergist will inject you with tiny amounts of venom. This will not cause an allergic reaction, but it will help your body build other defenses to the venom. In most cases, immunotherapy will desensitize your immune system to the venom. That means that the next time you get stung, you'll just get a welt like the rest of us. Because not all venoms are alike, your doctor will need to test you to determine which ones you're allergic to. You may need more than one series of injections to build your immunity to all the different venoms. We'll talk more about immunotherapy in chapter 11.

CHAPTER 7

Drug Allergies: The Wrong Prescription

Most of the time, drugs are our allies in the battle against disease. They help us recover from illness. They make our headaches disappear. They can help ease the symptoms of hay fever and stop asthma attacks before they start.

Once in a while, however, even the best of medicines can turn against us. They can cause all sorts of unexpected problems, from minor side effects like nausea and skin rashes to serious complications like high blood pressure. In rare cases, they can even cause allergic reactions. While most of these are mild, occasionally they're not. Severe allergic reactions to drugs can cause anaphylaxis, which may be life-threatening.

In this chapter, we'll explain how drug allergies start and how to tell the difference between minor side effects and potentially dangerous reactions. Then we'll explain what to do if you discover that you have a drug allergy. Taking a few simple precautions now can save you a lot of trouble later.

THE WRONG REACTION

It's not uncommon for people to have a bad reaction to drugs. In fact, as many as 30 percent of hospital patients have an unexpected or undesirable response to their medicines. But most of these responses are not related to allergies; they're called side effects or idiosyncratic responses. Only a fraction of drug reactions—as little as 6 percent—involve true allergic responses.

Most drug-allergy reactions occur when your immune system mistakenly creates antibodies against the drug. When molecules of the drug enter your body, the antibodies (made of immunoglobulin E) bind them to the outside of mast cells or basophils. The mast cells or basophils then release powerful chemicals like histamine, which cause typical allergic symptoms: runny nose, sneezing, hives, wheezing, and congestion—the same reactions you'd get from hay fever.

There's one difference between hay fever reactions and drug reactions. Unlike pollen or mold spores, drug molecules are often too small to grab the attention of the immune system. It's not until they combine with a part of your body—a blood cell, perhaps—that they are detected. The antibodies still deal with them the same way except that they drag the body cell into the action as well. As far as symptoms go, you can't usually tell the difference.

Drugs can also cause other types of allergic reactions. The reasons for this are quite complex. All you really need to know is that some drug reactions occur almost right away while others may not show up for 24 to 48 hours after exposure to the drug.

Years ago, a delayed allergic reaction called serum sickness was common. It often occurred when people received vaccines made from animal proteins. After the vaccine had been in the body for a week or more, the immune system would create antibodies to fight the foreign proteins. The antibodies would attach to the proteins in the vaccine in great numbers, then drift into lymph nodes, skin, and joints. The resulting inflammation from the allergic reaction caused sore joints and general body swelling. Although most vaccines are now made from nonanimal sources, serum sickness still occasionally develops in people after getting shots.

No matter what kind of allergy you have, you won't develop an allergic reaction to a drug until you've first become sensitized to it. This means you have to be exposed to it at least twice. The first time, your body creates the antibodies to fight the drug. The second time, you get a reaction. So if you react the first time you use a medicine, it's most likely an idiosyncratic response—not an allergic reaction.

Any drug can cause an allergic reaction. But some are more likely to do it than others. Penicillin and other antibiotics are the most common offenders. It's been estimated that as many as 10 percent of us may develop an allergy to these drugs. Other common allergy causers include sulfa-based drugs, barbiturates, anticonvulsant medications, local anesthetics like Novocain, and insulin (especially types of insulin made from animal sources).

Some people have a higher risk of developing drug allergies than others. Adults, for example, are more likely than children to have drug reactions. People who take large amounts of medications seem to develop more sensitivity than those who take less. And many drug allergies tend to be more common in people who use topical forms of medication. This may be because the skin is somehow more sensitive than the stomach and intestines, but it also may be due to the fact that topical forms are usually stronger than oral ones.

Aspirin and similar pain relievers can cause both allergic reactions and similar responses that mimic allergies. These nonallergic responses include swelling and possibly hives. Unfortunately, aspirin-like drugs are also a common trigger for asthma attacks. As many as 30 percent of children with asthma (and a similar number of adults who use steroids to treat their asthma) are sensitive to this effect.

DEALING WITH DRUG ALLERGIES

By now, this sentence should be burned into your brain: The best way to deal with allergies is to avoid the allergen. With drug allergies, that usually means switching to a different medicine. If you're allergic to penicillin, for example, your doctor will have to prescribe a different type of antibiotic. Things get a little complicated with drug allergies, however, because of something called **cross-reactivity**. Drugs with similar chemical properties may cause the same problems as the drug you're allergic to. This is a particular problem with penicillins and cephalosporins. If you're allergic to one penicillin, you'll almost certainly be allergic to all penicillin drugs.

If you've had a reaction while taking medicine, it's very important that you and your doctor find out exactly which drugs you're allergic to. A complete history is very important. You'll need to explain exactly what happened during your reaction: what type of symptoms you noticed, how soon they arrived, and how long they lasted. It's important to find out if you were exposed to the drug at an earlier date. If you developed a reaction the first time you used it, then you're probably not allergic to it.

A couple of tests can help, too. The most proven method is called an intradermal skin test. During this test, an allergist injects a tiny amount of the suspected drug allergen under your skin to check for a reaction. If you're allergic to it, you'll develop swelling and itching as from a mosquito bite within 15 to 20 minutes. A patch test also can identify drug allergies in some cases, especially for drugs that are applied to the skin, like topical antibiotics. Both tests are more complicated with drugs than with other allergens, however. That's because of the size of drug molecules. Some drugs need to combine with cells or proteins in your body before they're big enough to get the attention of your immune system. Without the body cells or proteins attached, the drug is harmless. Because the body cells or proteins aren't part of the patch or skin test, the test results may be falsely negative. It may take several sessions and some educated guesswork before your allergist is able to isolate your drug allergies.

Another choice for spotting drug allergies is called a provocational challenge. The allergist will give you a tiny dose of the suspected allergy causer to see if you have a reaction. It will be given to you in its usual form—by injection, orally, or on your skin. The dose at the beginning of the test is very small, as little as 1/100th or even 1/1000th of the typical dose. After a brief period (20 minutes to a couple of hours), you'll get a slightly higher dose. This process continues until you show signs of an allergic reaction. Sometimes it can take a day or longer until the allergist knows for certain whether you're allergic to the drug. The reason it takes so long is that the doses are small to prevent a serious reaction.

Once you know your drug allergy, it's best to just stop using the drug. That's not always possible, unfortunately. People with diabetes, for instance, can't stop using insulin just because they've had a bad reaction to it. In mild cases, you may need to take medications like antihistamines before taking the insulin or other drug you're allergic to. This can help ease or eliminate allergy symptoms. If that doesn't work, desensitization may be the answer. In this process, small amounts of the allergen are injected or swallowed into your body over the course of hours or a few days. Gradually, you'll build up a tolerance to the allergen.

One last word about drug allergies, and it's an important one. Drug allergies are a major cause of anaphylaxis. This is a rare but dangerous whole-body response that can cause the airways in your lungs to close down and a loss of blood pressure and consciousness. (These symptoms of anaphylactic shock are shown in the box on page 90.)

Anaphylactic reactions are most common in people who are allergic to penicillins and similar drugs. In fact, these drugs cause 97 percent of all deaths due to drug allergies. The best way to treat anaphylaxis is with a shot of epinephrine, a form of adrenaline. If you've had an anaphylactic reaction before, your doctor will probably give you an emergency injector that you can use until you make it to the emergency room. It's also a very good idea to wear an identification bracelet that warns doctors about your drug allergy. This can prevent serious problems in emergencies when you're treated by a doctor who doesn't know your history.

CHAPTER 8

Choosing an Allergist: When Allergies Are Out of Control

For most of us, allergies are a mild, seasonal problem. When pollen counts are high, we suffer. When pollen disappears, so do our symptoms.

If you belong to this group of occasional allergy sufferers, consider yourself lucky. Yes, you have allergies—and yes, they can make you miserable a couple of times each year. But with over-the-counter medication and a little avoidance, you'll do just fine. At most, you may need to see your regular doctor for a prescription medicine like a nonsedating antihistamine.

For some people, however, the road is a little rougher. Maybe you or your child has asthma. Maybe ragweed season makes your life completely unbearable. Perhaps you have frequent bad reactions after eating foods, or you're constantly breaking out in skin rashes. Or maybe you have symptoms that last all year long and defy all efforts to control them. That's when it's time to see an allergist—an allergy expert who can diagnose and treat your problem. Allergists perform tests and provide advice and medicine that may improve the quality of your life greatly. For people with severe allergies or asthma, a trip to the allergist can mean the difference between lifelong despair and being symptom-free.

WHEN AND WHY

Before you turn to the "A" section of the yellow pages, however, take stock of your situation. For starters, read the rest of this book. You'll find all sorts of advice on how to avoid allergens and choose over-the-counter medicines that may relieve your symptoms. An allergist will probably recommend that you try most of these tips before you take any tests or prescription drugs anyway.

It's also a good idea to visit your family doctor before looking up an allergist. Many times, a long talk with a general practitioner can solve your problems in a minimum amount of time—and for a minimum amount of money. With most managed care health insurance programs like HMOs, a visit to your primary care physician is required before you can get an appointment with an allergist.

This is not meant to scare you away from allergists. It's just practical advice. There are many situations in which visiting an allergist makes perfect sense. Here are some of them.

- ◆ When over-the-counter medications and simple allergen-avoidance techniques fail to relieve your symptoms

- When over-the-counter medications make you too drowsy to function normally or are not tolerable for another reason
- When allergies interfere with your daily life at work or school
- When your allergies have caused additional problems like recurring sinus infections, nasal polyps, or difficulty breathing
- When you have other medical conditions that interfere with ordinary allergy treatments, especially when you need to take medications that interact with allergy medicine
- When you suspect that you're allergic to something at work or school
- When you have suffered an anaphylactic reaction

People with asthma should visit an allergist at least once for a consultation. While primary care physicians can often help you manage your asthma properly, it's best to get an expert involved as well. Here are some indications that it's time to schedule an appointment with an allergist.

- When you or your child experiences asthma symptoms for the first time
- When you miss work or school because of asthma symptoms
- When asthma symptoms remain unstable despite the use of medication and avoidance procedures
- When you or your child visits an emergency room because of severe asthma symptoms
- When you or your child is hospitalized because of an asthma attack

There's one other case when it's advisable to see an allergist: when you think it's necessary. If you have honestly made your best attempt at controlling allergies or asthma—including proper use of medication and proper procedures for reducing allergens in your environment—and still gotten unacceptable results, by all means go ahead and call for an appointment. After all, it's your health, and you're the best judge of how allergies are affecting your life. If you think you can benefit from an allergist, there's no reason not to try.

When choosing an allergist, keep a couple of things in mind. First, you want the doctor to be certified by the American Board of Allergy and Immunology. This means that he or she has passed a qualifying examination and is up to date on the latest knowledge and techniques. Second, choose an allergist whose background fits your needs. Allergists are either internists or pediatricians. So if you're looking for an allergist for your young child, pick one who has a pediatric background. For you or another adult, choose the internist. All allergists must complete an additional two or three years of study to become certified specialists in allergic diseases.

Communication skills are almost as important as qualifications. Allergies can be complicated, so make sure your allergist is able—and willing—to take the time to explain what's happening. If you don't get the information you need, ask for it. If you still don't get it, ask for another allergist!

WHAT TO EXPECT

Your first visit to the allergist will probably involve a question-and-answer session. The allergist needs to know as much about you as possible so that he can develop a plan that's tailored to your needs. Be prepared to answer questions like the following:

+ Does either of your parents have allergies or asthma?
+ How long have you been feeling symptoms?
+ What kinds of symptoms do you have?
+ When and where do the symptoms show up?
+ How long do the symptoms last?
+ Do you have trouble sleeping because of allergy or asthma symptoms?
+ Do you or anyone in your house smoke?
+ Do you handle chemicals or dusts at work?
+ Are there any foods or medicines that you avoid? If so, why?
+ Do you have pets at home?
+ Are your symptoms worse at any particular time of the day or year?
+ What medications are you now using for allergies?
+ Do you have any other health problems?
+ Are you taking medication for another health condition?

The doctor probably will want to give you a brief physical examination, too. He will check inside your nose for signs of congestion, swelling, and polyps. Your mouth and throat may show signs of postnasal drainage. Your ears may have fluid in them. The doctor also will check for wheezing or congestion, plus skin rashes or hives. The answers you give to the questions, plus the physical signs you show, will help guide the allergist toward a diagnosis and method of treatment.

TESTS AND TREATMENTS TO AVOID

Allergy testing can be a confusing, frustrating process. And sometimes allergy sufferers will do just about anything to end their misery. Unfortunately, there are people out there who push unproven allergy tests and treatments on the public. We're not going to talk about these miracle "tests" and "cures" too much. But we will give you an idea of what to avoid.

Cytoxic tests sound like a good idea. They involve placing samples of your blood on a glass slide along with allergens. The slide is examined under a microscope to see if the blood reacts to the allergens. In practice, however, cytoxic testing is completely unreliable. Don't waste your time or your money on it.

You should also avoid tests called **IgG4 assays**. And never allow a doctor to do a procedure that involves injecting a small amount of your **urine** under your skin. It's a completely unproven process. Other people are pushing a **provocation and neutralization test**, which involves using small amounts of injected food allergens to both stimulate and then stop an allergic reaction. (We'll take another look at these on page 164.) Without getting too technical, we'll just say these tests don't work.

Another unproven theory holds that the fungus *Candida* causes all allergies. People are told to avoid eating foods that contain yeasts and molds, which are related to *Candida*. This is supposed to help the body fight off allergies—but, again, there's no proof that it works.

Not only are some treatments ineffective, but others are considered to be potentially harmful.

Finally, beware of **folk remedies** and **herbal medicines**. Many of the people who support these "cures" honestly believe in "natural" solutions to allergy. In time, some of their theories may prove to be legitimate. But at this point, none of them has been shown to be the least bit effective in identifying or eliminating allergies. (For more on therapies to steer clear of, see "Skip These Speculative Treatments" on page 164.)

It's highly unlikely that a reputable allergist will attempt to use any of these tests or treatments. If she does, simply refuse them—and find another allergist. Your health is too important to be left to unproven theories.

From there, it's on to the tests. An allergist has many tests available—everything from skin pricks to double-blind food challenges. Which tests you get depend on the nature and the severity of your symptoms. But they're all designed to identify your specific allergy or allergies. Here's an overview of the common tests that you may encounter.

Skin tests. There are two broad categories of skin tests. One checks for immediate allergies caused by immunoglobulin E (IgE) antibodies, such as hay fever, most food and drug sensitivity, and insect stings. The second type of test is for allergies that aren't caused by IgE antibodies, such as delayed reactions to poison ivy or nickel.

IgE tests are done in one of two ways. The first is called a skin-prick test. The allergist will place a highly diluted amount of an allergen on your skin, then poke the skin gently with a needle. This pushes the allergens under the skin, where they react with IgE antibodies on skin mast cells. After about 20 minutes, the allergist will check the area to see how large a bump (called a wheal) or how much redness (called a flare) has developed. He'll compare this to another site on your skin where he has placed a saltwater solution. If you have a larger wheal or flare where the allergen was injected, then you're sensitive to that substance.

The only problem with this test is that people taking antihistamines or steroids won't have much of a reaction to the allergen, which can confuse the results. You'll need to be off the medications for a period of time (three days to three months, depending on the antihistamine) before the test results are valid.

The second procedure is called an intracutaneous or intradermal test. Instead of placing the allergen on the surface of the skin, the allergist uses a syringe to inject it under the surface. This test can identify weak allergic sensitivities better than the skin-prick test. But it has drawbacks. For one thing, it involves a needle, which bothers some people. More important, there's a greater risk of an anaphylactic reaction when the allergen is injected under the skin. As with the skin-prick test, the intracutaneous test is affected by the use of antihistamines and medications.

If your doctor suspects you have a contact skin allergy to a cosmetic or drug, you'll probably get another type of skin test: a patch test. Unlike other allergy skin tests, this one is often performed by a dermatologist (a skin specialist) instead of an allergist. The doctor will place one or more (sometimes many more) allergen-containing patches on your skin. The patches usually stay on for about 48 hours, then are removed. The doctor then looks for signs of allergic reactions, especially blisters such as you might get from poison ivy. These tests are very useful for determining whether you have a true skin allergy or a nonallergic sensitivity to a substance like formaldehyde. There's a lot of educated guesswork in reading the results of patch tests, and experience counts for a lot. Steroid medication sometimes interferes with patch test results.

Blood tests. If your allergist is unsure whether you're actually suffering from an allergy, you may be tested for the presence of IgE antibodies. These are the antibodies that grab on to allergens as they enter your body and trigger the release of chemicals like histamine. Almost everyone has some IgE antibodies, but people with allergies, asthma, and eczema usually have far more than normal. This is a simple test, but it has limits. For example, it's not specific to an allergen. While the test may show that you have high levels of IgE antibodies, it won't be able to tell exactly which allergen most of the antibodies were created to fight. In fact, you could have parasites, which also cause high IgE levels.

A second type of blood test is allergen-specific. If your doctor suspects that you are allergic to a certain substance, your antibodies can be tested against that particular substance. This test is called the radioallergosorbent test, or RAST. The doctor takes a sample of blood, then removes the blood cells, leaving a clear fluid called serum. This fluid is then placed in a machine that counts the different types of IgE antibodies. It's superior to the first blood test because it can tell you specifically which allergens your body has made IgE antibodies to fight. But it's far from perfect. For starters, it takes longer than a skin-prick test and is usually no more accurate. And, as with all allergy tests, the results may be misleading. Just because you test positive for antibodies to a certain allergen doesn't mean that the allergen is the one causing your problems. It may be another allergen that hasn't been tested for.

Food tests. If your allergist thinks you may have a food allergy, there are two main tests available. Both of them are time-consuming, but they can pinpoint exactly which foods have allergens that your body reacts to. It's important that you identify the source of serious food reactions, since there's a risk of anaphylactic reactions (see "Symptoms of Anaphylactic Shock" on page 90) if you eat the offending food.

The first test is called an elimination diet. This involves removing certain foods from your diet for a while to see whether your symptoms go away. It sounds like a simple idea. If you're allergic to shellfish only, then you won't have an allergic reaction unless you eat crabs, lobster, or shrimp. (Mussels, clams, and oysters are much less often implicated.) But in practice it's often more difficult than that. Many times, people are allergic to proteins that appear in many different foods or food additives. Unless you have a precise record of what you did and didn't eat, the test may not be of value. An elimination diet can take weeks to identify the allergen, but the results are certainly worth the wait.

The second food test is called a double-blind food challenge. Many allergists consider this the gold standard of food testing. This test involves taking gel capsules that contain proteins commonly found in foods. Some of these capsules, however, are filled with inert sugars that won't cause a reaction under any circumstances. They are called placebos. They're used to make sure that the test is not influenced by expectations. Sometimes people can start feeling sick to their stomach if they just think about eating a certain food. Because the capsules aren't identifiable by your doctor, even he doesn't know which ones are real and which ones are placebos. That's so that he won't be able to give you any subtle body-language hints about what's in the capsules. He won't misinterpret the results based on his biases.

After recording your reactions to the capsules, the allergist will check the results against a written record to see which proteins you may be allergic to. Again, this process can take a few weeks since you may have to start with low doses for safety reasons, and many foods may need to be evaluated, each at multiple doses.

Drug tests. Since patch and skin-prick tests are often unreliable for identifying drug allergies, the best method is a graded-dose challenge (also called a provocational challenge). The allergist will give you minute doses of the drug that is suspected of causing a reaction. After a period ranging from about 20 minutes to a few hours, the allergist will give a slightly more potent dose of the drug. This continues until you show signs of an allergic reaction or safely reach a full dose. The whole process can take a day or longer. The provocational challenge also is used in some cases of food-allergy testing.

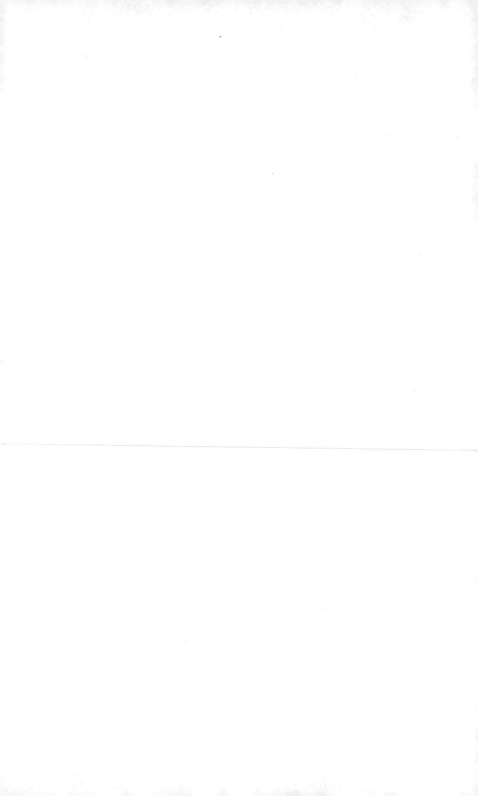

CHAPTER 9

Cleaning House: Your Allergy-Proof Environment

Quiz time! When it comes to cleaning house, do you:

    A. Vacuum and scrub?
    B. Sweep it under the rug?
    C. Skip it and shrug?

If you chose "A," congratulations. You're helping to make your house an allergy-free zone. Experts believe that you can reduce the number of allergens in the home by controlling dust, mold, and other particles that can trigger an allergic reaction or asthma attack.

In this chapter, we'll talk about specific steps you can take in every room of the house, plus some tricks you can use outside to keep your exposure as low as possible. Some of them are easy, like washing bed linens in hotter water. Others can be more complicated—and more expensive—like buying a special vacuum cleaner system to filter out fine particles of dust.

How far you go with this is really up to you. But if you answered "C" in the quiz, chances are that making a few changes in your weekly routine might make a big difference. A little more effort around the house each day may help reduce your allergy symptoms all year long.

THE USUAL SUSPECTS

If you're allergic to pollen only, then allergy season is pretty well defined. When pollen is in the air, you suffer. When it's not, you don't. But the story is different when you're allergic to things that last year-round. These can cause perennial allergic rhinitis and asthma—allergies that give you grief no matter what the calendar says.

There are four big culprits in year-round allergies: dust mites, mold, pet dander, and cockroaches. Every one of them may be present in your house. Let's take a look.

Dust mites. These are the number-one household allergy problem. Dust mites are tiny creatures that are related to spiders, ticks, and chiggers. They can't be seen with the naked eye, and they feed off the skin we shed every day. Their waste products contain proteins that can cause allergic reactions when sensitive people breathe them. They accumulate in bedding, carpets, and upholstered furniture. About 1 person in 10 appears to be sensitive to dust mite excretions, and nearly 90 percent of children with asthma are affected.

Live mite populations are usually highest in mid-summer and decline in the winter. But that doesn't make life any easier in the winter. You spend more time inside during the cold months, and forced-air heat can spread mite allergens all over the house.

Mold. These organisms ask for just two things: moisture and darkness. Once they find them, molds merrily reproduce. They do this by creating spores.

These lightweight cells float on the slightest breeze in search of other places to grow. Unfortunately, these spores contain proteins that can cause any number of allergy symptoms.

Mold grows easily on shower doors. Damp carpeting is a favorite spot. So are windowsills. And humidifiers. And damp firewood that you bring in from outdoors. Even damp wallpaper, shoes, and refrigerators often serve as mold colonies.

Pet dander. Dogs and cats shed more than just hair. They also slough off skin, which is called dander. The proteins in this dander can be a major source of problems. Cats are especially troublesome because the same protein also gets spread through their saliva when they wash themselves.

While many people believe that getting rid of a dog or cat is the only way to solve pet allergies, things may not have to be so extreme. You can declare some rooms—especially bedrooms—off-limits to your pets. Washing your pet frequently, perhaps as often as once a week, can help keep dander under control. And regular brushing outside can remove dander from your pet's skin before it has a chance to fall on the carpet or furniture.

Unfortunately, just about any pet with fur will eventually cause problems for a person who's allergic to dander. You'll be better off with some goldfish or a bird than you will with guinea pigs, hamsters, gerbils, ferrets, or any other mammal.

Roaches. Droppings and remains from cockroaches are a major household trigger for allergy and asthma. This problem is especially severe in urban areas, where roaches can easily spread from one apartment to another.

Extermination and thorough cleaning to remove food sources are usually needed to control this problem.

ALLERGY "STUFF"

While mold, dust mites, cockroaches, and pet dander are the main indoor allergy triggers, many other substances also make things worse. Smoke from cigarettes, pipes, cigars, and even fireplaces can irritate the sinuses of allergy sufferers and may increase the likelihood that small children will develop allergic sensitivities. High-odor products like paints, solvents, and perfumes also are potential troublemakers for allergy sufferers.

ROOMS FOR IMPROVEMENT

We spend more time in our homes than anywhere else. We sleep eight hours a day in our bedrooms. We eat meals in our dining rooms. We watch television or read in the den. We do homework at our kitchen tables and wash clothes in our basements. And every morning we take showers and brush our teeth in our bathrooms.

Every room in your house presents different challenges. Here's a room-by-room plan to make your house as allergen-free as possible.

Bedrooms. You spend up to one-third of your life in the bedroom. If any room needs to be allergen-free, this is the place.

Let's start with the bed itself. Over time, skin cells can work their way through the bedding and into the mattress, making it a favorite spot for dust mites, as you might imagine. That's why it's very important to encase the mattress in an airtight cover. These come in plastic, which are the cheapest, and polyurethane-treated cloth.

THE SNEEZE-PROOF BEDROOM

You spend more time in your bedroom than anywhere else. So it pays to keep allergens as far away as possible. Here are 10 tips.

1. Use an air conditioner.
2. Keep windows closed.
3. Install wood flooring or low-pile carpeting.
4. Buy a HEPA filter.
5. Keep the door closed.
6. Place filters over air vents.
7. Keep the room clutter-free.
8. Keep clothes in the closet.
9. Wash bedding weekly at least.
10. Use dust-proof covers for pillows and mattress.

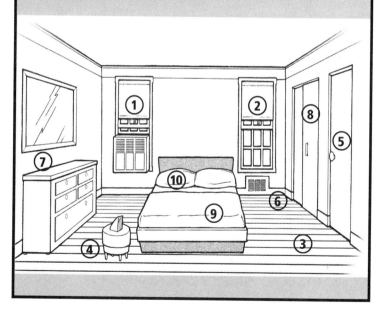

The polyurethane types tend to "breathe" a bit more, making them more comfortable to sleep on. These products are available in many retail stores. Before you put on the cover, make sure you vacuum the mattress thoroughly to remove as much dust as possible.

The same treatment works for your pillows, too. Many people assume that feather pillows are more likely to cause allergic reactions. A small study from New Zealand, however, found that they are no worse than synthetic-filled pillows. But since it's a good idea to wash your pillows every 7 to 10 days, you'll probably find it easier to buy a pillow stuffed with polyester or another synthetic material. Foam rubber pillows are not recommended.

Like pillows, all bed coverings need to be cleaned every 7 to 10 days. The key here is to use hot water that is at least 130 degrees Fahrenheit (55 degrees Celsius). It's a good idea to use blankets and bedspreads that can be machine washed, since you're going to be cleaning them often. Dry cleaning is more expensive than washing and may not be as effective at mite control. Japanese researchers found that hot-water washing removes about 95 percent of mite allergens, while dry cleaning takes care of only about 70 percent.

Now, the flooring. Carpets, particularly those laid over concrete floors, are like giant dust mite condominiums. They're usually slightly moist and are hard to clean deeply. It's an excellent idea to remove wall-to-wall carpeting in your bedroom. Replace it with linoleum or hardwood. Either surface is much easier to clean than carpet, and mites don't survive well on them.

The floor doesn't have to be bare. You can use throw rugs to keep your feet warm. Just make sure you can machine wash them to remove dust mite allergens. One Australian research team found that placing rugs upside-down on a hot outdoor surface for four hours killed just about all mites and their eggs.

Remember how Mom used to get on you about picking up your room? Well, she had a point. Clutter in bedrooms creates more places for dust to gather. Make sure your bedroom isn't loaded with knickknacks, including wall hangings and stuffed animals. Dust furniture and windowsills at least once a week, too.

It's important to mention humidity: Mites and mold love it. That means that the drier your room, the less likely you are to have allergy problems. Of course, home heating systems can make rooms almost unbearably dry in the winter. If you think you have to add humidity to a room, make sure the level doesn't rise past 40 or 50 percent. This will keep dust mites down. It's important to keep your humidifier extremely clean, however. Dirty filters are breeding grounds for mold. And rinse the water receptacle with a mild white vinegar solution every week.

Hot-air heating systems not only make air dry, but also stir up and carry dust and mold around the house. It's important to keep furnace filters clean and to vacuum the ductwork several times a year. If your allergies are severe, you can try taping a piece of cheesecloth over the ducts in your bedroom. This will act as an additional filter, although it may cut down somewhat on airflow.

OUTSIDE CONTROLS

While you don't have much control over allergens that drift in from your neighbors' yards, you can at least take charge of what happens on your own property. Here are a few hints.

- Keep your rain gutters clean. This keeps mold from growing on rotting leaves.
- Keep wet firewood away from the house. Again, this helps control mold.
- Pay someone else to do the yardwork. The next-door neighbor's son can save you all sorts of sneezing by cutting your grass, pulling your weeds, and raking your leaves. Of course, this isn't free. If you insist on doing things yourself, at least wear a mask that filters pollen and mold. You can get one at the hardware store.
- Keep your grass short. If it's two inches or shorter, it won't be able to pollinate.
- Stay out of the yard in the late morning (10 a.m. to noon), when pollen counts are often highest.
- Change your clothes and shower immediately after finishing your chores. This will keep you from breathing pollen and mold that are on your clothes and body.

The plants you choose for landscaping can be very important. Here's a brief list of plants that are generally allergen-free, since they are bee-pollinated and have heavy pollen that can't float as freely through the air.

Trees: Pear, yew, fir, fruited mulberry, magnolia, cherry, dogwood

Shrubs: Azaleas, boxwood, oleander, hibiscus, yucca

Plants: Geraniums, crocuses, hyacinths, daffodils, roses, bougainvillea, ferns, orchids, lilies, petunias, vinca, begonia, lavender, cacti
Other plants, however, release lighter pollens that can cause allergic reactions in many people:
Trees: Maple, birch, ash, elm, willow, walnut, cottonwood, olive, nonfruiting mulberry, cypress
Shrubs: Privet, juniper
Plants/grasses: Bluegrass, Bermuda grass, amaranth, sorrel, timothy

While a large green lawn is part of the American Dream, it can be a true allergic nightmare. If you're sensitive to grass, you may want to consider cutting back on the size of your lawn. You can expand your flower beds—just make sure you plant flowers and shrubs from the preceding "good" list. And you can plant ground-covering plants on other parts of your property. Plants like vinca and ferns are beautiful, cover bare spots quickly, and won't give you the sniffles.

In the summertime, air conditioners can be a godsend to allergy sufferers. They help keep air dry and clear of airborne particles. If your house does not have central air-conditioning, consider buying a window unit for the bedroom. As with humidifiers, make sure the filters are clean so that mold doesn't get a foothold in your bedroom.

Here's another helpful hint: Keep the windows closed. Your room may be warm in the summertime, but opening your windows can let in every pollen, spore, and other allergens that are floating in the air. Fans aren't great since they can stir up dust and other particles that have settled in your bedroom. Again, air-conditioning is your best bet. It helps keep air cool, dry, and clean.

By the way, if you take all these precautions and still wake up during the night with a stuffed-up nose, it could be due to a late-phase response. This means that you were exposed to an allergen earlier in the day and are only now experiencing symptoms. For example, you may breathe in pollen on your commute home and suffer the consequences at night, even though your room is clean and sealed from the outdoors.

One last note about the bedroom. If you or a family member has a severe allergy or asthma problem, the bedroom may be a great place for a HEPA—high-efficiency particle-arresting—air filter. These are super-fine filters that can take most allergens out of the air. Good models can be expensive (starting at $100 or more), but they can be well worth the cost if you have serious problems. Make sure that the machine you choose has enough power to recirculate the air in your bedroom at least five times an hour. Remember that opening a door or window will nullify the effects of a room air filter.

Bathrooms. Mold is the big problem here because bathrooms provide the two things mold needs most: moisture and darkness.

Think about it. You take a nice steamy shower, towel off, then close the bathroom door and turn off the lights. All that moisture settles in corners, on the wallpaper, and on the floor. Pretty soon, you've got a regular mold factory going.

The key to fighting allergens in the bathroom is to make the place inhospitable to mold. First, make sure there's a fan that vents humid air to the outside. If there's no vent, then crack a window to allow moisture to escape. And if there's no window, leave the door open when you're done and think about putting a dehumidifier in the room. Even though the room will still be dark when you leave, mold won't get established if there's no moisture.

Second, clean surfaces like walls, floors, and shower stalls with antimold products. There are scores of them on supermarket shelves these days, or you can make your own. Just mix one tablespoon of chlorine bleach with one quart of water.

Kitchen. Again, mold and cockroaches are the major problems. Mold thrives in a couple of places. First is the refrigerator. Most have water pans that catch drips before they hit the floor. If you don't clean them regularly, you're just asking for mold. Use the same bleach solution you used in the bathroom when cleaning the water pans.

The second kitchen problem is cockroaches. Roaches are especially attracted to kitchen areas because of the supply of food and water. The single best way to limit roach problems is to keep food tightly covered. Also, keep counters and sinks as clean as possible. And don't forget to keep a lid on your garbage.

If you still have trouble controlling roaches, consider hiring an exterminator. If you decide to try killing them yourself, use traps, poison baits, gels, or paste. Boric acid is a common and effective ingredient. If you decide to spray for roaches, make sure the person suffering from allergies or asthma stays out of the area until the fumes and odor go away. These could be triggers for another allergy attack.

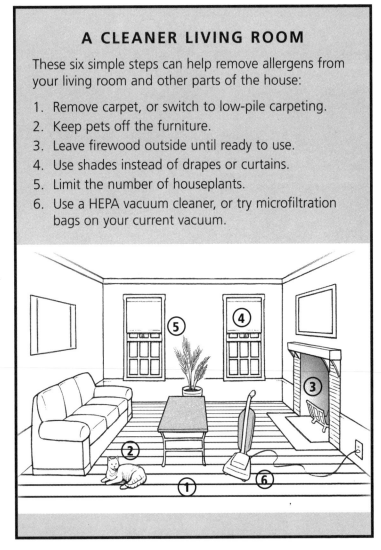

A CLEANER LIVING ROOM

These six simple steps can help remove allergens from your living room and other parts of the house:

1. Remove carpet, or switch to low-pile carpeting.
2. Keep pets off the furniture.
3. Leave firewood outside until ready to use.
4. Use shades instead of drapes or curtains.
5. Limit the number of houseplants.
6. Use a HEPA vacuum cleaner, or try microfiltration bags on your current vacuum.

Living room. Dust and pet dander are the big problems here. If you have wall-to-wall carpeting, consider pulling it up and replacing it with throw rugs and a hardwood or linoleum floor. If that's not an option, try to use a low-pile carpet instead of a shag style. Low-pile carpets are easier to keep clean with regular vacuuming.

Speaking of vacuuming, it may be time to put your old Hoover out to pasture. Models that have regular dust bags aren't doing your allergies any favors. In fact, dust, mites, and mite residue can pass right through the bag and spread around the room as you run the vacuum cleaner. You have two options. The first is to stop using regular bags and switch to microfiltration bags. These are usually double-thick, so they trap dust particles better. And many of them have an electrostatic charge that holds on to dust. It's getting easier to find these bags in regular stores, although you can't get them for every model. If you have trouble finding one that fits, contact the manufacturer of your vacuum cleaner and ask for help.

This won't work for every vacuum cleaner. Some have leaky seals and worn hoses that just can't do the job properly anymore. If that's the case with your old workhorse, consider buying a vacuum cleaner with a true HEPA filter. These are more expensive than regular vacuum cleaners (starting at $500 or more), but they're the best thing going for people with dust mite allergies. As an alternative, sensitive people can wear a dust mask when running the vacuum cleaner.

There's a good deal of controversy right now about whether treating carpets with chemicals to kill dust mites is an effective way to control allergies. Two types are on the market. The most common formula contains benzyl benzoate. It's available in a powder that you sprinkle on carpets. While some tests have shown that the powder helps kill mites, others have found little effect on mite populations. One thing is clear. If you're going to use it, it must be reapplied frequently, probably once a month.

The other chemical is tannic acid. It's applied in spray form, in either a 1 percent or 3 percent solution. Again, the test results have not been conclusive about whether it really helps reduce mite allergens. For now, the best solution remains proper vacuuming or, better yet, removing the carpet altogether.

Here are a few additional tips for the living room.

- Keep pets off the furniture so their dander doesn't settle into the upholstery.
- Use shades instead of heavy cloth drapes. They're easier to clean.
- Don't store firewood inside. It can be moldy. In fact, people with allergies and asthma are often sensitive to wood smoke, so keep fires to a minimum.
- A HEPA filter will help clean the air further. But it's less clear whether respiratory symptoms are significantly reduced by using a filtering device. If you decide to invest in one, make sure that it's large enough to handle the square footage of the room; the machine's room-size rating is usually listed on the box.
- Go easy on the houseplants. Wet soil is an ideal breeding spot for mold.

Closets. Dust clings to clothes. Ideally, handle them the same way you handle bedsheets: wash them in hot water (at least 130 degrees Fahrenheit). Unfortunately, not all fabrics can take hot-water washes. So make sure that most of your wardrobe can take the beating. Read the labels to make sure hot water is okay.

Wet shoes and boots also can be a mold source. Before you put them in the closet, make sure they're dry.

Basement. Watch out for mold. Many basements are damp, so a dehumidifier will help. If your furnace is in the basement, make sure that you change the air filters at least once a month. And if your clothes dryer is in the basement, make sure it has a vent to the outside. Otherwise, you'll be spewing warm, moist air back into the house.

By the way, clothes dryers can be helpful for people with allergies. That's because clothes that hang outside can pick up pollen and mold spores from the air. When you put on the clothes, the pollen gets disturbed—and you breathe it in.

CHAPTER 10

Drug Therapy: The Next Step

Allergens are sneaky things. You can clean your house top to bottom, keep the windows closed, run the air conditioner, wash the clothes in hot water, install a HEPA (high-efficiency, particle-arresting) filter, cover your sheets and pillows—and allergies are still going to slip through once in a while. Even if your home is airtight, there are still times you'll come into contact with allergens—pollens in the air, say, or mold at work or dander from someone's cat.

That's when it's time to call on the second line of defense against allergies: medications. The combination of avoiding allergens and drug treatment is enough to get most people through even the toughest allergy season. In many cases, over-the-counter medications will take care of your symptoms without a trip to the doctor. In this chapter, we'll look mainly at drugs used to treat hay fever and perennial allergic rhinitis. You'll find information on drugs used specifically for asthma and skin allergies in the chapters covering those conditions.

There are three main categories of anti-allergy drugs: antihistamines, decongestants, and corticosteroids. They attack allergic reactions in different ways and counteract different symptoms. They also have different side effects. Let's take a look.

ANTIHISTAMINES

Doctors have been treating allergies with antihistamines for more than 50 years. Antihistamines have proven to be an effective way to head off allergic symptoms before they start. They're especially useful for stopping sneezing, itching, and rhinorrhea (the medical term for runny nose). They won't give you much relief from nasal congestion, however; for that you'll need another type of medicine.

Antihistamines work by blocking the action of histamine, a powerful chemical that is contained in mast cells and basophils. When allergens appear in your body, antibodies located on the surfaces of these cells grab on to them. The antibodies, thinking they have intercepted a harmful invader instead of a simple little protein, signal the mast cells or basophils to release their load. Out comes histamine, along with a number of other chemicals. Their job is to eliminate the allergens. But in the process, they cause all sorts of irritating problems, like sneezing, congestion, hives, and runny noses.

Once released, histamine flows through the body looking for places to work. It usually latches onto cells that make up the lining of blood vessels. Histamine slips inside these cells and starts killing "invaders" (as well as the cells themselves). To get into the cells, however, it first has to bind onto special moorings called **histamine receptors**. These are located on the outside of the cells. The histamine fits into the receptor like a key into a lock. When you have allergies, of course,

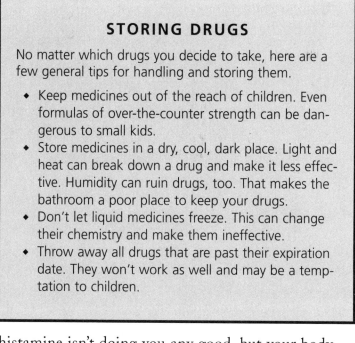

STORING DRUGS

No matter which drugs you decide to take, here are a few general tips for handling and storing them.

- Keep medicines out of the reach of children. Even formulas of over-the-counter strength can be dangerous to small kids.
- Store medicines in a dry, cool, dark place. Light and heat can break down a drug and make it less effective. Humidity can ruin drugs, too. That makes the bathroom a poor place to keep your drugs.
- Don't let liquid medicines freeze. This can change their chemistry and make them ineffective.
- Throw away all drugs that are past their expiration date. They won't work as well and may be a temptation to children.

histamine isn't doing you any good, but your body doesn't know this.

There's a limit to how much histamine can latch onto each body cell. Once all the cell's receptors are full, that's it. The remaining histamine must continue to float around looking for an unused receptor.

That's where antihistamines come in. As the name suggests, they block the effects of histamine so you don't develop allergic symptoms. Antihistamines work because they have the same sort of "key" as histamine. When you take an antihistamine, the medicine makes its way from your digestive system into your bloodstream. It seeks out histamine receptors on the blood vessel cells and grabs hold.

Unlike histamine, antihistamines don't try to activate the cell and cause problems; they just hang around and take up space. When histamine comes floating past, in search of a place to dock, it sees a "No Vacancy" sign on the cell receptors, which are filled up with antihistamine molecules. With nowhere to go and nothing to do, the histamine eventually breaks down and gets reabsorbed by your body. And the mast cells and basophils stop releasing additional histamine when they sense that none of it is being used. It's a dirty little trick that antihistamines pull, but it works remarkably well. As many as 8 people in 10 get good results from antihistamines.

The problem with antihistamines is that they're much less useful when an allergic reaction is already under way. Once it's released, histamine gets to work in a hurry. By the time you notice symptoms like a runny nose or hives, histamine has already grabbed onto the receptors and started its business. If you take antihistamines at this point, they're the ones that are going to be floating around looking at "No Vacancy" signs. They may help a little, but most of the damage is already done by this point.

So the key to using antihistamines is anticipation. When you know that pollen or mold counts are high, it's best to take antihistamines about half an hour before you go outside. That gives the medicine a chance to work before your body releases histamine. The same thing goes if you're visiting someone with a cat or dog. Take the medication shortly before you leave home, and your symptoms may be greatly reduced.

There are two major kinds of antihistamines. The first are known as sedating antihistamines. These are older medications that work well, but cause drowsiness in about 25 percent of people who take them. This is because the antihistamines work their way from the bloodstream into your brain, where they can slow some basic brain functions. In addition to feeling drowsy or groggy, many people report that they have trouble concentrating.

Interestingly, many people who suffer from these side effects don't even realize it. One study found that many people felt they weren't the least bit tired or groggy when, in fact, their psychomotor skills were impaired significantly. For this reason, it's extremely important to follow the directions when taking the medication. If they say not to drive or operate machinery while using it, heed the warning. And don't drink alcohol while you're taking antihistamines. Alcohol is a depressant that can increase the sedating characteristics of the drug. Fortunately, the grogginess eases for many people after they've been using sedating antihistamines for a while.

Other side effects from sedating antihistamines include dryness in the mouth, nose, and eyes. In rare cases, people may have insomnia, dizziness, constipation, diarrhea, or difficult urination. Some of these side effects can be serious, so report them to your doctor immediately. Sedating antihistamines are the only kind available in over-the-counter formulas.

In the 1980s, drug manufacturers developed a new class of antihistamines, the "second-generation" or nonsedating, antihistamines. These are no more effective than the original antihistamines in warding off symptoms from an allergic reaction. But they have a couple of advantages over their older cousins. First, they rarely cause drowsiness. That's because the antihistamines don't get into the brain. They just attach to the blood vessels and do their work where they should. For this reason, they can be used by people who need to drive, operate machinery, or concentrate hard at work or school.

The second advantage is that many of these drugs come in a time-release version. The older antihistamines start losing their effectiveness within a few hours, so you have to take the medicine every 4 to 6 hours. But the second-generation drugs continue to work for up to a full day. Most people have to take only one or two doses every 24 hours, which simplifies things quite a bit. In addition, the nonsedating antihistamines are less likely to cause dryness in the nose, eyes, and mouth.

Of course, with the good sometimes comes some bad. Second-generation antihistamines are available by prescription only, and generic versions are not yet available. This makes them more expensive than the sedating antihistamines.

More important, some second-generation antihistamines may cause serious heart problems in some people. The main drug in question is terfenadine. Its brand name is Seldane or Seldane-D (which also contains a decongestant). The Food and Drug Administration (FDA) has reported that terfenadine can lead to irregular heartbeats and even fatal heart rhythm problems in people who are taking other drugs to treat illnesses not related to allergies. These drugs include the following:

- Some antibiotics (erythromycin, clarithromycin, and azithromycin)
- Antifungal preparations that include ketoconazole and itraconazole

- AIDS medicines such as Crixivan, Norvir, Invirase, and Viracept
- The heartburn drug Propulsid
- The blood pressure drug Posicor
- Serotonin reuptake inhibitors such as Luvox, Zoloft, and Serzone
- The asthma drug Zyflo

In addition, the FDA warns that drinking grapefruit juice while taking terfenadine can be dangerous because it may increase the drug's effects. Although the FDA approved the drug in 1985, the manufacturer has now decided to remove Seldane and Seldane-D from the market. Other drugs can perform the same tasks without the risks, including fexofenadine, known as "Son of Seldane" or Allegra.

Another second-generation antihistamine, astemizole (Hismanal), has come under similar scrutiny. Some research has found that Hismanal may cause some of the same problems as Seldane, but so far the FDA has not moved to take this product off the market. Again, talk to your doctor if you have concerns.

None of this is meant to scare you away from using antihistamines. For the vast majority of people, they're very safe and extremely effective against allergy symptoms. It's just that you should always be careful about taking medications, no matter what they're for. Sometimes they have unintended effects. For this reason, you should consult your doctor before taking any antihistamine, especially if you

- Are pregnant or are trying to become pregnant
- Are breast-feeding a child

♦ Use antidepressant medications known as MAO (monoamine oxidase) inhibitors

♦ Have glaucoma or an enlarged prostate gland (In these cases, second-generation antihistamines are usually preferred.)

DECONGESTANTS

Antihistamines can take away the runny nose, itching, and sneezing. But they don't do much for one of the most uncomfortable allergy symptoms: a stuffed-up nose. That's where decongestants come in. They can help open up your sinuses and get you breathing easy—sometimes within minutes.

Most people assume that their noses feel stopped up because they're filled with mucus. But that's only part of the trouble. When an allergic reaction strikes, your body responds by inflaming your sinuses, causing them to swell. It does this in part to make the nose an uninviting place for germs and other bad guys to live (remember, your body thinks that the harmless allergen is actually one of these undesirable invaders). The swelling you feel is caused by a greater flow of blood to the nose. Of course, when the inside of your nose swells up, there's less room for air to pass. And that makes it harder to fill your lungs.

Decongestants ease this inflammation by constricting the smooth muscles around your blood vessels. This makes them narrower, so less blood flows through. Less blood in the nose means less swelling. And less swelling means you can keep your mouth closed and still get enough air to breathe.

Because they each do things the other one can't, decongestants and antihistamines make a very powerful pair. In fact, many prescription and over-the-counter allergy medicines contain both types of drugs. The combination has one other advantage. Over-the-counter antihistamines can make you drowsy, but for many people, decongestants are stimulating because they tend to increase blood pressure temporarily. Obviously, that's not good for everyone. But it can help counteract the effects of antihistamines and keep you awake during the day.

Unlike antihistamines, decongestants work even if you take them after an allergic reaction begins or when nonallergic causes like cold air and smoke have produced nasal congestion. They'll help unstuff a nose that's been swollen shut for hours. So if you inhale an allergen before you can take your medication, there's still a good chance your nose will open up for you later.

Decongestants are available in two forms: oral tablets and nasal sprays. The inhalers can be wonderful when used wisely. They deliver the medicine directly into your nose, where you need it most. Pills, on the other hand, first go into the stomach, then work their way into the bloodstream and nervous system before they do you any good. That can take an hour or more, while nasal inhalers get to work within minutes.

As often happens, however, there's a price to pay for this speed. It's called the **rebound effect**. Nasal sprays shouldn't be used for more than a few days in a row. After that, they can actually make your sinuses swell up more when the medicine begins to wear off (usually within a couple of hours). In effect, your nose becomes dependent on the inhaler medicine. Once you've started this reaction—called chemical rhinitis—stopping it can be a long and uncomfortable process. By all means, use decongestant nasal inhalers for immediate relief. Just be careful not to overdo things. After you have things under control (at most, a couple of days), it's a good idea to switch to oral decongestants.

Decongestants aren't free of side effects either. While their stimulating quality might be good to balance anti-histamines, it can get out of hand. Some people who take decongestants report that they feel restless, nervous, or jittery. For this reason, it's a good idea to go easy on other stimulants like coffee, tea, colas, diet pills, and "pep" pills like Vivarin. Many times, your body learns to adjust to this stimulating effect. So you may feel less antsy after you've been taking decongestants for a couple of weeks or so.

Overstimulation may be a minor nuisance for some people. But for others, it can be dangerous. This is especially true for people who have high blood pressure. Sometimes decongestants interfere with medicines that are designed to keep blood vessels open wide. People with heart problems may not tolerate decongestants well either.

Pregnant and breast-feeding women should consult their doctors before taking decongestants. The same goes for people with diabetes.

CORTICOSTEROIDS

In the battle against allergy symptoms, corticosteroids are the undisputed heavyweight champions. They are terrific at blocking inflammation, which means they're good for relieving stuffed-up noses, hives, and bronchial swelling. They seem to halt many allergic reactions before they start. They're also good for blocking delayed allergic reactions, which can come hours or even days after the initial attack. And they're widely effective; almost everyone who uses them gets good results.

Corticosteroids for fighting hay fever come in three forms: nasal sprays, oral tablets, and injections. Nasal sprays are usually the first choice. They deliver the medicine only to the part of your body that needs it most. There's little, if any, concern about side effects. About all you might encounter is a little irritation in your nose and maybe an occasional nosebleed. You can use nasal corticosteroid sprays to treat hay fever, perennial (year-round) rhinitis, and sinusitis.

Nasal corticosteroids usually are used to treat moderate allergy symptoms and are prescribed only when a patient doesn't respond well to an antihistamine/decongestant combination. Increasingly, however, doctors are prescribing corticosteroid nasal sprays as a first option. People usually don't build up a tolerance to the sprays, as they sometimes do with particular types of antihistamines and decongestants. This means you can stick with the same medicine all the time. Here's another bonus: You need to use the inhaler only once or twice a day. This makes it a lot easier to remember when to take your medicine, so you're more likely to follow your doctor's orders.

Nasal corticosteroid sprays are available in a water-based solution and as a gas-driven powder. They're equally effective, although some people tolerate one type better than the other. While the water-based sprays can help moisturize your nasal linings, they may also increase nasal drip. While the powders don't have that problem, they sometimes have an odor that people don't care for. At this point, all nasal corticosteroids are available by prescription only.

If you don't get enough relief from a nasal corticosteroid spray, your doctor may try combining it with an antihistamine/decongestant formula. But if you're one of those people who suffers severe symptoms during the height of allergy season, you may need even stronger medicine. Oral or injected corticosteroids are about as strong as you can get (in fact, about the only time you should consider an injected steroid is if you're hospitalized). They work throughout your body to battle allergic reactions, and they're usually very effective. The problem is that you can use them only for a little while. If you take them for more than a few weeks at a time, oral corticosteroids such as prednisone can cause any number of undesirable side effects. These can include fluid retention, muscle weakness, loss of muscle tissue, thinning of the skin, ulcers and other digestive system troubles, cataracts, osteoporosis, and slowed growth in children. The side effects can be serious, but most people won't have problems when they use the drugs for a short time. For some people, they're the only answer to allergy symptoms that make life unbearable.

CROMOLYN SODIUM

This drug is much better known for its ability to ward off asthma attacks. But some doctors are using cromolyn sodium to treat hay fever and perennial rhinitis. The drug appears to work by making it harder for mast cells to release their toxic load of histamine and other chemicals. Since these chemicals cause most allergy symptoms, keeping them bottled up is a very effective way to control reactions to allergens. The problem with cromolyn sodium is that it has absolutely no effect once a reaction is under way. It's strictly a preemptive weapon; taking it even a few minutes after exposure to an allergen is pretty much a waste of time. Once you start taking it, you'll have to continue using the medication through the entire allergy season. Missing even one dose can cause your allergies to flare.

Cromolyn sodium is used as a nasal spray in people with hay fever. (For those with asthma, it's delivered directly to the lungs.) It probably has fewer side effects than any other allergy drug; some people may notice an occasional headache or a burning sensation in their nostrils, but that's about it. Almost anyone can take cromolyn sodium—even pregnant women and kids. The only real downside is that you probably will need to use the nasal spray four or more times a day for it to be effective.

Nedocromil is very similar to cromolyn sodium. It's also used mainly for asthma prevention, but is often prescribed for people with allergic asthma. Like cromolyn, nedocromil will not prevent an allergy attack once it starts. You may need to take the drug every day for at least two weeks before it works best to prevent asthma symptoms.

EYEDROPS

Oral allergy medications like antihistamines and decongestants will often take care of watery, red, itchy eyes. But if your eye symptoms become too severe, there are plenty of eyedrops available. Before you take them, however, first try flushing your eyes with cool water. This can relieve symptoms and wash allergens like pollen out of your eyes.

Many eyedrops on the market today contain drugs similar to nasal decongestants. They're called vasoconstrictors, which means they reduce swelling and redness by making your blood vessels narrower. Like nasal decongestants, they can have a rebound effect. If you use them too much, your eyes will become dependent on the medicine. When you stop using the drops, your eyes will turn even more red than they were before. So if you want to use eyedrops, do so sparingly. Wait until your symptoms are at their worst. And don't use the drops for more than about three days in a row.

Many eyedrops now contain antihistamines. While the decongestants handle redness, the antihistamines go to work on the itching and tears. Many eyedrops combine antihistamines and decongestants to take care of both problems at once. Again, though, you have to watch for the rebound effect.

CHOOSING THE RIGHT DRUG

It's bad enough to be cloudy-headed from hay fever. Then you have to go to the drugstore and choose the right medication. If you have a prescription, things are pretty cut-and-dried. But if your doctor recommends an over-the-counter formula, the choices can be truly dizzying.

Let's try to make things as simple as possible. Before you go to the store, decide what kind of medicine you need. Are you sneezing? Teary-eyed? Is your nose running? Then you're looking for an antihistamine. If your nose is stuffed up, on the other hand, you're going to need a decongestant. If you have symptoms that call for both types of drugs, there are combination antihistamine/decongestant products.

Be prepared to take a little time before you pick a product. That's because you'll have to read the labels to make sure the products are right for you. If you don't want to take a pill every four hours, make sure you choose a product that you need to take only once or twice a day. If you can't afford to be drowsy during the day, then avoid over-the-counter antihistamines, all of which are sedating. If you or your child can't take pills well, consider a liquid form or nasal spray.

And if you have questions about which medicine to choose, by all means talk to the pharmacist. Better yet, consult your doctor before you go to the store. A little knowledgeable, friendly advice can save you all kinds of aggravation and indecision.

The list of allergy-fighting medications changes constantly. That makes it difficult to create a complete list of over-the-counter and prescription products. But a sampling of brand names and products that you're likely to encounter is shown in the boxes on the following pages.

We need to add a couple of warnings for people with special medication needs. First, children: Under no circumstances should you give children adult-formula allergy medications. This is especially important with over-the-counter antihistamines, which can make children very drowsy. There are child-strength allergy

COMMON MEDICATIONS
FOR ALLERGY SYMPTOMS

GENERIC NAME   *BRAND NAME(S)*

Sedating Antihistamines

By Prescription Only
Cetirizine	Reactine, Zyrtec
Chlorpheniramine	Chlor-Tripolin
Clemastine	Tavist
Cyproheptadine	Periactin
Diphenhydramine	Diphenadryl, Benoject, Wehdryl
Hydroxyzine	Atarax, Vistaril
Tripelennamine	Pyribenzamine (PBZ)

Nonprescription Formulas (Over-the-Counter)
Brompheniramine	Dimetane
Chlorpheniramine	Chlor-Trimeton
Clemastine	Tavist (also in prescription formula)
Diphenhydramine	Benadryl

Nonsedating Antihistamines

By Prescription Only
Astemizole	Hismanal
Azatadine	Optimine
Fexofenadine	Allegra
Loratadine	Claritin

Decongestants

Oral Formulas (Over-the-Counter)
Pseudoephedrine	Drixoral Non-Drowsy, Sudafed, Children's Sudafed

Nasal Sprays (Over-the-Counter)
Ephedrine	Vicks Vatronol
Oxymetazoline	Afrin, Dristan Long-Acting, Neo-Synephrine Maximum Strength, Vicks Sinex Long-Acting
Phenylephrine	Dristan Fast-Acting, Neo-Synephrine (pediatric, mild, regular, and extra strength formulas), Vicks Sinex

ALLERGY MEDICATIONS
AND THEIR ACTIVE INGREDIENTS

Brand Name   *Active Ingredient(s)*

Antihistamine/Decongestant Combinations

By Prescription Only

Allegra-D	Fexofenadine, pseudoephedrine
Claritin-D	Loratadine, pseudoephedrine

Over-the-Counter

Actifed	Triprolidine, pseudoephedrine
Allerest	Chlorpheniramine, pseudoephedrine
Benadryl Decongestant	Diphenhydramine, pseudoephedrine
Chlor-Trimetron	Chlorpheniramine, pseudoephedrine
Contac	Chlorpheniramine, pseudoephedrine
Dimetane Decongestant	Chlorpheniramine, pseudoephedrine
Dimetapp	Brompheniramine, phenylpropanolamine
Drixoral Cold and Allergy	Dexbrompheniramine, phenylpropanolamine
Sudafed Plus	Chlorpheniramine, pseudoephedrine
Tavist-D	Clemastine, phenylpropanolamine
Triaminic	Chlorpheniramine, phenylpropanolamine
Vicks Dayquil	Brompheniramine, phenylpropanolamine

Cromolyn Sodium

Over-the-Counter

Nasalcrom	Cromolyn sodium

Eyedrops

By Prescription Only

Livostin	Levocabastine
Patanol	Olopatadine

Over-the-Counter, for redness (decongestant only)

Clear Eyes ACR	Naphazoline, zinc sulfate
Murine Plus	Tetrahydrozoline, povidone
Visine A.C.	Tetrahydrozoline, zinc sulfate

Brand Name	Active Ingredient(s)
Eyedrops	
Over-the-Counter, for redness, watering, and itching (decongestant and antihistamine)	
Alcon	
Naphcon A	Naphazoline, pheniramine
Bausch & Lomb	
Opcon-A	Naphazoline, pheniramine
Vasocon-A	Naphazoline, antazoline

formulas on the market today, many of which come in easy-to-take liquid forms. But it's a good idea to talk to your pediatrician before giving children any medication for allergies.

Older people may be strongly affected by sedating antihistamines. If these over-the-counter drugs make you too drowsy, talk to your doctor about prescribing a nonsedating antihistamine instead. And always be careful about mixing over-the-counter allergy medications with drugs that you take for other conditions. Some drug combinations can be dangerous. As always, read labels carefully and talk to your doctor if you have any doubts or questions.

We're going to turn our attention now to the next step in allergy prevention: allergy shots. They're the third piece of the allergy-fighting puzzle. If you have made an honest effort to reduce your exposure to allergens—and if over-the-counter and prescription drugs haven't given you the relief you need—allergy shots may help. They're not perfect and they're not for everyone. But they might make a difference for you.

CHAPTER 11

Immunotherapy: A Shot at Long-Term Relief

To this point, we've focused mainly on two trusty ways to handle allergies. The first is avoidance: don't breathe, eat, or touch any allergens; keep your house spotless; and tread lightly around insects like honeybees and fire ants. The second is medication. Many drugs can help relieve allergy symptoms, as well as more serious problems like asthma.

In this chapter, we'll look at a third option—immunotherapy, better known as allergy shots. It's attractive because it offers one thing that the other methods can't: the possibility that you can become desensitized to pollens, mold spores, and other allergens.

Immunotherapy is not a cure for allergies. While it can greatly reduce your risk of having an allergic reaction, it's far from foolproof. It's not for everyone, either. Some people are better candidates than others, and some allergens are easier to deal with than others. Immunotherapy is a long process as well. It can take years of treatments to get the best results. It involves dozens and dozens of shots and can be expensive. And the tolerance you build to the allergen may not last forever.

Of course, compared with the alternatives—severe or constant allergic symptoms—immunotherapy can be a very attractive option. Let's take a closer look at how immunotherapy works.

STOPPING THE RESPONSE

Let's review how most allergic reactions occur. When a harmless protein in pollen, a mold spore, or another allergen enters your body, it encounters your immune system. Your immune system mistakes it for a dangerous intruder and creates antibodies to fight it. The next time you're exposed to the allergen, the antibodies (which are made of immunoglobulin E, or IgE) grab it and bind it to a mast cell or basophil. These cells then release powerful chemicals like histamines that kill the allergen, and in the process they give you symptoms ranging from a stuffy nose to anaphylaxis.

Immunotherapy short-circuits this process. A doctor injects you with tiny, diluted amounts of an allergen. This grabs the attention of a different antibody—immunoglobulin G (IgG). This antibody gets tricked into thinking that the allergen is actually an invading germ. To fight the "germ" in the future, your body creates more IgG. The antibodies intercept the allergen and neutralize it before it has a chance to reach the IgE antibodies that cause those dreaded allergic symptoms.

Over time, your body creates enough IgG antibodies to fight off a full-fledged invasion of allergens. They wipe out the allergen, leaving IgE antibodies with nothing to do. Eventually, the IgE antibodies die off, and you lose your sensitivity to the allergen.

Doctors have been working to perfect immunotherapy for most of this century. They've come a long way since the early 1900s, but the treatment still has many short-comings.

It doesn't always work. Immunotherapy can be a lifesaver for those with dangerous allergies to stinging insects. Studies have found that immunotherapy can help up to 98 percent of people develop at least limited immunity to venom from bees, wasps, and hornets. Success rates are also very high (80 percent and higher) for airborne allergens like ragweed, some tree and grass pollens, house dust, and mold. Immunotherapy may also help those who are allergic to cat and dog dander.

But immunotherapy has not proven successful against other major allergens. Skin allergies to poison ivy, poison oak, and nickel, for example, don't respond to immunotherapy because they're not IgE-related responses. Neither are many food reactions. And you won't get relief from sensitivities to things like feathers or strong chemicals, perfume, or smoke, either.

The list of allergies that immunotherapy can help is growing. Researchers are learning how to standardize extracts of many allergens, which will allow better treatment eventually. But for now, there are some allergens that you're just going to have to learn to avoid.

It's not for everybody. Before an allergist will even consider you a candidate for immunotherapy, you have to meet certain criteria.

- Are your allergy symptoms severe enough to warrant a treatment that can last for years? Do these symptoms have a major impact on your everyday life?

- Is it clear that what you react to on skin or RAST (radioallergosorbent tests) actually causes symptoms when it enters your body?
- Have you taken all the necessary steps to reduce contact with your allergens? Have you installed allergen-proof covers on your pillows and mattresses? Do you close your windows at night? Do you wash your clothes and bed linens in hot water?
- Are you allergic to something that's unavoidable? If you are allergic to cats, for example, you're best advised to find a new home for your pet. But if you are a veterinarian, that's a different story. You see cats up close and personal every day, and you're going to need some help.
- Have you missed time at work or school because of your allergies?
- Do you still have allergy symptoms even though you're taking large doses of medication?

And that's just the first cut. Even when you meet these standards, your doctor will need to know a few more things.

- Do you have a medical condition that might interfere with treatment for a reaction to an allergy injection? If you have high unstable angina or have recently had a heart attack, you may not be able to tolerate an epinephrine shot. People who take beta-blockers for high blood pressure or heart problems shouldn't have immunotherapy.
- Do you follow doctor's orders? Immunotherapy takes a long-term commitment. If you have trouble remembering to take pills, or have a history of

stopping treatments on your own, immunotherapy isn't for you. It requires a lot of perseverance.

♦ Can you communicate with your doctor? Anaphylaxis is a possible side effect of immunotherapy. It's rare, but it can be deadly for people who aren't able to tell their doctor that they're feeling the signs of anaphylactic shock. This means that young children (under four years of age or so), people with mental or psychological problems, and others who have trouble getting their point across don't make good candidates.

Immunotherapy has been used for years to help people with severe asthma. Even though asthma isn't a purely allergic reaction, many times the triggers for asthma attacks are allergens like mold and pollens. Many studies have found that immunotherapy can be effective for asthma. But a recent study found that it may not benefit children who are already receiving proper asthma treatments like modern medication and avoidance therapy. These results have started a hot debate in the field of allergy research, and there's been no agreement on how to proceed. For now, discuss the issue with your child's doctor—and don't stop immunotherapy treatments unless the allergist agrees.

WHAT TO EXPECT

Once you're established as a good candidate for immunotherapy, the shots can begin. Many people are allergic to more than one substance, so the shot may include several allergens at once. The allergens are greatly diluted to start—usually by about 1,000:1 but sometimes as high as 10,000:1.

SKIP THESE SPECULATIVE TREATMENTS

Allergies can make people so miserable that they'll go to almost any length to find relief. Unfortunately, there are lots of unproven or even dangerous treatments out there, each one claiming to offer the cure you've been looking for.

Here are a few treatments you're better off skipping.

Neutralization therapy. People who believe in this treatment claim that taking a small amount of an allergen can stimulate the body to ward off symptoms brought on by full exposure to the allergen. Extracts of the allergen are taken by injection or by placing a drop under your tongue. People are instructed to take the extract when they start to feel allergy symptoms or before they think they're going to be exposed to the allergen.

While it sounds a little like regular immunotherapy, the treatment is unproven and can be dangerous, especially if used for food allergy.

Autologous urine injections. Believe it or not, some people claim that injecting yourself with an extract of your own urine can ward off allergies. The theory is that urine contains a substance called proteose that eliminates allergic reactions. Again, there's no evidence that this method works. And some experts fear that substances found in urine could prove dangerous when placed back in your body.

Diet and vitamin therapies. According to proponents, eating complex combinations of food or taking a combined variety of vitamins, amino acids, and other substances can hamper the body's allergic response. This remains unproven and can even be harmful to people who make radical changes in their diet or take too many vitamins.

This is altogether different from making simple dietary changes to avoid food allergies. Avoiding foods that cause reactions is a proven way to deal with food allergies.

Homeopathy. People who believe in homeopathy claim that ingesting minute amounts of food or plant extracts will prevent allergic reactions. While homeopathy has grown in popularity, there simply is no hard evidence that it helps at all.

After the shot, you'll sit in the doctor's office for a while, usually about 20 minutes because there's a chance you might have a reaction to the shot. It is something that you're allergic to, after all. At some point during your treatments, you'll probably have a mild, local reaction to the shot—possibly swelling near the injection site. If other symptoms develop after you leave the office, it's important to call your doctor and tell her about the reaction. Cold packs and antihistamines may help relieve the local swelling, but make sure you advise your doctor before you do anything.

In approximately 10 percent of cases, a general, or systemic, reaction may occur. This may take the form of hives far away from the injection site. Or it could be more serious. Anaphylaxis, which may cause tightness in the chest, difficulty breathing, dizziness, swelling of the tongue and lips, and a feeling of impending doom, can also occur. (See "Symptoms of Anaphylactic Shock" box on page 90.) This is more likely to happen when you first start treatment or get a refill of your injection solutions. It's extremely important that you get your immunotherapy treatments at an office or clinic that's equipped to handle anaphylaxis. Be sure to ask before you get a shot.

Immunotherapy is very safe, but there are risks. A few Americans die each year after having an anaphylactic reaction to a shot. That works out to about one fatality for every three million shots.

You'll usually get one or two shots a week for at least 16 to 20 weeks. If things go well, you'll start to feel a little relief within four to six months. But that's not always the case. Sometimes it can take two to three years to get maximum relief. Your allergist will evaluate you at least once a year to make sure that you are showing some progress.

Depending on how your body reacts, your doctor will slowly increase the amount of allergen in each injection. Over the course of months, you'll work your way up to a dilution that's 1,000 times stronger than the first dilution—a real sign that you're gaining tolerance to the allergen. The process is not always smooth, however. You're likely to reach a point somewhere in the treatment where your body has an adverse reaction to the allergen. Then the allergist will probably slow down the increases, giving your body a chance to build tolerance at its own pace.

Once you are able to handle the top dilution, you're in maintenance mode. The shots will continue on a regular basis (every two to four weeks), but the dosage will remain at about that level. How long you keep up the maintenance shots is up to your immune system.

AN ALTERNATIVE METHOD

The continuous injection treatment we've just described is the method most doctors prefer because it usually works the best. But there is an alternative. This method is called rush immunotherapy. This is a fast process that can give you limited tolerance to an allergen in a matter of days. It's typically used for people who need protection from insect stings fast. The process may involve several injections each day, given as quickly as one hour apart. Because you build up the doses rapidly, there's an increased risk of an allergic reaction. In fact, you may be asked to take antihistamines and corticosteroids as you're getting the shots, which will help stop reactions before they start. Because of the higher risk, it's vital that you only get these treatments from a doctor who has experience with rush immunotherapy—at a location that's able to handle severe reactions like anaphylaxis.

Most allergists will wait until you go a full year without allergy symptoms, then decide whether it's time to stop the treatments. This whole process can take four to six years.

Immunotherapy doesn't work for everyone. If you're not going to get any benefit from the treatments, there's no point in continuing them. That's especially important if money is an issue, because immunotherapy can be costly. Shots for the first year can run as high as $1,000. It gets a little cheaper in later years, since you'll probably be receiving fewer treatments. There's another way to look at the cost, however. If successful, immunotherapy could significantly cut your costs for medications to treat the allergy symptoms that you no longer feel.

After the injections stop, you'll probably enjoy a period with few allergy symptoms. This could last months or years—or maybe forever. For many people, mild allergy symptoms eventually will return. Remember that your immune system still thinks the allergen is a foreign invader. When allergens manage to slip past the IgG antibodies created by the immunotherapy, your body will respond by creating IgE antibodies, the ones that cause symptoms. The good news is that the symptoms are usually far milder than before and can be treated with medication. If symptoms grow worse, you may need to restart the allergy shots until things get under control again.

As you can see, immunotherapy is far from perfect. So before you start treatments, think hard about whether the whole process will be worth it. Unless your symptoms are severe enough to interfere with your health or everyday life, immunotherapy may not be for you.

Of course, researchers are always looking for ways to improve allergy treatments. Later we'll look at what may lie in the future for you and millions of others— including genuine vaccines that may actually make you immune to allergens.

CHAPTER 12

The Future of Allergy Treatment

Every year, doctors and researchers discover exciting new ways to treat asthma, allergy symptoms, and allergic reactions. The medicines available today are far better than they were a decade ago, and there's no reason to think they won't be better yet 10 years from now.

But what about the ultimate quest—a cure for allergies and asthma? Will it someday be possible to get an injection or take a pill and never have to worry about hay fever or asthma or anaphylaxis again? Will eating shellfish no longer cause hives? Will we be able to picnic in a patch of poison ivy and not get a single blister?

The answer is a definite . . . maybe. Allergies are complex. The world is full of allergens, and all of them behave differently. It may never be possible to block all allergic reactions with a single treatment. But we may someday be able to knock out allergens one at a time with vaccines or other treatments. Some of the early research in this direction has been promising, yet there's still a lot of work to be done. Let's take a look at some of the treatments now under development.

PEPTIDE VACCINES

This is a new spin on an old treatment: immunotherapy. In current practice, doctors give people a series of injections containing tiny amounts of an allergen. This allows you to build up partial resistance to the allergen. But the process can take years to be effective and often has to be repeated.

Now, researchers are trying to use tiny pieces of the allergens, called peptides, to create the same type of resistance. A peptide is a small chain of amino acids, which are the building blocks of protein (remember, most allergens are proteins). By using only a piece of the allergen, the hope is to create tolerance without any of the risks or side effects of standard immunotherapy. Early research shows that the peptides are not as likely to cause allergic reactions when they enter the body through an injection. Such reactions are very common with today's immunotherapy, and sometimes can lead to serious problems.

There could be other advantages to the peptide vaccines. For one thing, they may be less expensive than immunotherapy, since it may be easier to synthesize peptides than it is to isolate the tiny amounts of natural allergens that are now used. Second, the vaccines may work more quickly. Testing is now under way for peptide vaccines that treat allergies to ragweed pollen, dust mites, pollens from several grasses and trees, and even cat dander.

IgE SUPPRESSION

Immunoglobulin E, or IgE, is a key factor in many allergies. Antibodies made of IgE bind with allergens, triggering the release of histamines and other chemicals that start the allergic reactions for hay fever, food allergies, insect stings, and more. So cutting off the supply of IgE in the body seems like a logical way to stop reactions before they start.

There may be several ways to accomplish this. One is to create a substance that combines with IgE antibodies and makes them unavailable to hook onto mast cells. Until they attach to mast cells, IgE antibodies can't do any harm. Once they're attached, however, they can signal the mast cell to release its load of chemicals. The substance that's been developed to link with the IgE antibodies is called a monoclonal antibody. It's a genetically engineered substance that's still in the testing stages. So far, it has shown promise in fighting hay fever and dust mite allergies and, more recently, allergic asthma.

Specialized T lymphocytes determine the amount of IgE antibodies produced by the body. Using altered allergens or peptide fragments may be a way to alter the T lymphocytes to "help" without triggering an allergic reaction. There's one big problem, however: How do you alter only T cells that limit IgE production? After all, your body needs other antibodies, like IgG and IgM, to fight infections. Limiting their production could make you vulnerable to other, more serious diseases.

In fact, stopping IgE production may not be such a great thing, anyway. We don't know exactly why the body creates IgE antibodies, but it must do it for some good reason. It doesn't make sense that the body would make a substance that only triggers useless harmful allergic reactions. Many researchers believe that IgE antibodies help fight off attacks from parasites. So eliminating or cutting back on IgE antibodies could make us more vulnerable to them.

DISABLING MAST CELLS

If IgE antibodies are the trigger of allergic reactions, mast cells are the loaded gun. When the IgE antibodies hook onto an allergen, they stimulate the mast cells to release their chemical content, which causes the runny nose, sneezing, watery eyes, hives, and nasal congestion that you feel when you have an allergic reaction. If researchers can find a way to block the release of these chemicals, it would stifle the reaction.

Some experts believe that a substance called Syk (pronounced "sick") is involved in releasing the mast cell's chemicals. Syk is a protein that's contained in the mast cell. Researchers are trying to develop a molecule that would bind with Syk and prevent it from doing its job. The advantage of this approach, which is still very early in the development process, is that you wouldn't have to build resistance to an allergen since the mast cell wouldn't operate even when the IgE antibodies tell it to.

STOPPING OTHER CHEMICALS

Although it's the biggest player in allergic reactions, histamine is not the only bad guy. Many other substances play a role. Prostaglandins are one. There are many kinds of prostaglandins, and they serve many useful functions in your body. But one type of prostaglandin can make the smooth muscles around your lung airways tighten up, causing bronchospasms and making asthma attacks worse. Another type makes blood vessels dilate, or grow

BODY SYSTEM FACTORS

Experts have long believed that stress and other psychological factors can play a big role in how well your immune system works. No one is quite sure how or why this happens. But it's now becoming apparent that the immune system is linked closely to two other networks in your body: the endocrine system and the central nervous system.

The endocrine system creates hormones. The thymus and pituitary glands, for example, are part of the endocrine system. The central nervous system includes your brain and nerves that send impulses through the body. Scientists are now finding that receptors on many cells in these systems are designed to fit with parts of the immune system and vice versa. This means what happens in your brain might play a big role in what happens in your lungs and nasal passages. This may be why stress and emotional upset can trigger or aggravate asthma attacks and other allergic symptoms.

It's way too early to predict how these links between body systems could help yield a cure for allergies. But it's an exciting and wide-open field at this point.

wider. At the same time, it makes the vessels more permeable, meaning that more fluid can flow from the blood into surrounding tissues, causing swelling. It even makes you more sensitive to the pain of swollen tissues.

Leukotrienes are also involved in allergic reactions. Like some prostaglandins, leukotrienes can lead to constricted airways in the lungs. Other types seem to be responsible for attracting inflammatory cells to the site of an allergic reaction. This makes the reaction worse by increasing the amount of chemicals and cells available to fight the harmless allergen.

One day, stopping allergic reactions may be as easy as taking a pill or getting a single shot. But we're not there yet. Research will continue, and life will no doubt improve for the millions of us who dread hay fever season or live in fear of bee stings or food allergies. For now, an ounce of prevention remains the best medicine. Until we figure out how to stop allergies before they start, the only sure way to avoid reactions is to avoid allergens. Because what you don't breathe—or touch or eat—can't hurt you.

APPENDIX

GENERAL INFORMATION

These organizations offer information, pamphlets, and other materials about allergies and asthma.

Allergy Research Group
400 Preda Street
Post Office Box 480
San Leandro, CA 94577
Telephone: (800) 545-9960

American Academy of Allergy, Asthma, and Immunology
611 East Wells Street
Milwaukee, WI 53202
Telephone: (414) 272-6071; (800) 822-2762
This organization offers the United States Pollen Calendar, which lists average bloom times for a number of allergy-causing plants. The Academy also offers a free national referral service. Callers can receive names, addresses, and telephone numbers of allergists who have been certified by the American Board of Allergy and Immunology.

**American College of Allergy, Asthma &
Immunology**
85 West Algonquin Road
Suite 550
Arlington Heights, IL 60005
Telephone: (800) 842-7777
*This organization also offers a free national referral
service.*

American Lung Association
432 Park Avenue South
New York, NY 10016
Telephone: (212) 889-3370
*The Association provides general information on
asthma and other respiratory diseases. It also runs
smoking cessation programs.*

Food Allergy Network
4744 Holly Avenue
Fairfax, VA 22030
Telephone: (703) 691-3179
*The network offers guidelines on food allergies for
patients, parents, and teachers.*

National Asthma Education Program
4733 Bethesda Avenue
Suite 350
Bethesda, MD 20814
Telephone: (301) 495-4484

National Institute of Allergy and Infectious Diseases
31 Center Drive
MSC 2520
Building 31, Room 7 A 50
Bethesda, MD 20892-2520
Telephone: (301) 496-5717

SUPPORT GROUPS

Allergy and Asthma Network/Mothers of Asthmatics, Inc.
3554 Chain Bridge Road
Suite 2000
Fairfax, VA 22030
Telephone: (800) 878-4403

Asthma and Allergy Foundation of America
1125 15th Street NW
Suite 502
Washington, D.C. 20005
Telephone: (202) 466-7643
This is a lay support organization for allergy patients and their families. It offers a wide variety of services and has local and state chapters as well.

Parents of Asthmatic/Allergic Children
1412 Marathon Drive
Fort Collins, CO 80524
Telephone: (303) 842-7395

INTERNET RESOURCES

Internet websites can offer fast, free, and valuable information about allergies and asthma. Be warned, however, that the Internet is a big place and not all of the sites you'll run across will be legitimate. Also, Internet addresses tend to change. The following is a list of reputable websites run by recognized national organizations.

Allergy, Asthma & Immunology Online
http://www.allergy.mcg.edu
This site is run by the American College of Allergy, Asthma & Immunology.

American Academy of Allergy, Asthma and Immunology
http://www.aaaai.org
This site, as well as Allergy, Asthma & Immunology, is run by professional associations of asthma and allergy specialists. Both offer a wide range of general information for allergy and asthma sufferers.

American Lung Association
http://www.lungusa.org
This site contains dozens of documents about allergies, asthma, and other lung-related conditions. You'll find news articles, medical and legislative updates, and fact sheets.

Allergy and Asthma Network/Mothers of Asthmatics, Inc.

http://www.podi.com/health/aanma

This is an award-winning site that offers information on asthma, including frequently asked questions, product updates, and lists of asthma specialists nationwide.

Asthma and Allergy Foundation of America

http://www.aafa.org

This site contains games, educational materials, how-to instructions, and lists of frequently asked questions. A valuable site for children and teenagers.

The Food Allergy Network

http://www.foodallergy.org

This comprehensive website offers daily tips, updates, product information, and a newsletter about food allergies.

InteliHealth

http://www.intelihealth.com

The online partner to Johns Hopkins Health offers comprehensive information on asthma and allergy and features timely updates on new drugs and research discoveries.

PRODUCTS

Environmental Protection Agency
Public Information Service
401 M Street, SW
Washington, D.C. 20460
Telephone: (800) 438-4318
Provides information on air-filtering devices.